THE TRUTH ABOUT ANXIETY AND DEPRESSION

SECOND EDITION

Robert N. Golden, M.D.
University of Wisconsin–Madison
General Editor

Fred L. Peterson, Ph.D.
University of Texas–Austin
General Editor

Heather Denkmire
Principal Author

John V. Perritano
Contributing Author

William Kane, Ph.D.
University of New Mexico
Adviser to the First Edition

Mark J. Kittleson, Ph.D.
Southern Illinois University
Adviser to the First Edition

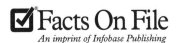

Facts On File
An imprint of Infobase Publishing

The Truth About Anxiety and Depression, Second Edition

Facts On File, Inc.
An imprint of Infobase Publishing
132 West 31st Street
New York NY 10001

Library of Congress Cataloging-in-Publication Data
Denkmire, Heather.
  The truth about anxiety and depression / Heather Denkmire, principal author ; John Perritano, contributing author ; Robert N. Golden, general editor, Fred L. Peterson, general editor. — 2nd ed.
     p. cm.
  Includes bibliographical references and index.
  ISBN-13: 978-0-8160-7643-7 (hardcover : alk. paper)
  ISBN-10: 0-8160-7643-X (hardcover : alk. paper) 1. Anxiety—Popular works.
2. Depression, Mental—Popular works. I. Perritano, John. II. Golden, Robert N. III. Peterson, Fred (Fred L.) IV. Title.
RC531.T78 2010   616.85'22—dc22
          2010005461

Text design by David Strelecky
Composition by Erika K. Arroyo
Cover printed by Art Print, Taylor, PA
Book printed and bound by Maple Press, York, PA
Date printed: November 2010
Printed in the United States of America

10 9 8 7 6 5 4 3 2 1

This book is printed on acid-free paper.

CONTENTS

LIST OF ILLUSTRATIONS

PREFACE

The Truth About series—updated and expanded to include 20 volumes—seeks to identify the most pressing health issues and social challenges confronting our nation's youth. Adolescence is the period between the onset of puberty and the attainment of adulthood. Adolescence is also a time of storm, stress, and risk-taking for many young people. During adolescence, a person's health is influenced by biological, psychological, and social factors, all of which interact with one's environment—family, peers, school, and community. It is a time when teenagers experience profound changes.

With the latest available statistics and new insights that have emerged from ongoing research, the Truth About series seeks to help young people build a foundation of information as they face some of the challenges that will affect their health and well-being. These challenges include high-risk behaviors, such as drinking, smoking, and other drug use; sexual behaviors that can lead to adolescent pregnancy and sexually transmitted diseases (STDs), such as HIV/AIDS; mental-health concerns, such as depression and suicide; learning disorders and disabilities, which are often associated with school failures and school dropouts; serious family problems, including domestic violence and abuse; and lifestyle factors, which increase adolescents' risk for noncommunicable diseases, such as diabetes and cardiovascular disease, among others.

Broader underlying factors also influence adolescent health. These include socioeconomic circumstances, such as poverty, available health care, and the political and social situations in which young people live. Although these factors can negatively affect adolescent health and well-being, as well as school performance, many of these negative health outcomes are preventable with the proper knowledge and information.

With prevention in mind, the writers and editors of each topical volume in the Truth About series have tried to provide cutting-edge information that is supported by research and scientific evidence. Vital facts are presented that inform youth about the challenges experienced during adolescence, while special features seek to dispel common myths and misconceptions. Some of the main topics explored include abuse, alcohol, death and dying, divorce, drugs, eating disorders, family life, fear and depression, rape, sexual behavior and unplanned pregnancy, smoking, and violence. All volumes discuss risk-taking behaviors and their consequences, healthy choices, prevention, available treatments, and where to get help.

In this new edition of the series, we also have added eight new titles in areas of increasing significance to today's youth. ADHD, or attention-deficit/hyperactivity disorder, and learning disorders are diagnosed with increasing frequency, and many students have observed or know of classmates receiving treatment for these conditions, even if they have not themselves received this diagnosis. Gambling is gaining currency in our culture, as casinos open and expand in many parts of the country, and the Internet offers easy access for this addictive behavior. Another consequence of our increasingly "online" society, unfortunately, is the presence of online predators. Environmental hazards represent yet another danger, and it is important to provide unbiased information about this topic to our youth. Suicide, which for many years has been a "silent epidemic," is now gaining recognition as a major public health problem throughout the life span, including the teenage and young adult years. We now also offer an overview of illness and disease in a volume that includes the major conditions of particular interest and concern to youth. In addition to illness, however, it is essential to emphasize health and its promotion, and this is especially apparent in the volumes on physical fitness and stress management.

It is our intent that each book serve as an accessible, authoritative resource that young people can turn to for accurate and meaningful answers to their specific questions. The series can help them research particular problems and provide an up-to-date evidence base. It is also designed with parents, teachers, and counselors in mind so that they have a reliable resource that they can share with youth who seek their guidance.

Finally, we have tried to provide unbiased facts rather than subjective opinions. Our goal is to help elevate the health of the public with an emphasis on its most precious component—our youth. As young people face the challenges of an increasingly complex world, we as educators want them to be armed with the most powerful weapon available—knowledge.

Robert N. Golden, M.D.
Fred L. Peterson, Ph.D.
General Editors

HOW TO USE THIS BOOK

NOTE TO STUDENTS

Knowledge is power. By possessing knowledge you have the ability to make decisions, ask follow-up questions, and know where to go to obtain more information. In the world of health, that is power! That is the purpose of this book—to provide you the power you need to obtain unbiased, accurate information and *The Truth About Fear and Depression.*

Topics in each volume of the Truth About series are arranged in alphabetical order, from A to Z. Each of these entries defines its topic and explains in detail the particular issue. At the end of most entries are cross-references to related topics. A list of all topics by letter can be found in the table of contents or at the back of the book in the index.

How have these books been compiled? First, the publisher worked with me to identify some of the country's leading authorities on key issues in health education. These individuals were asked to identify some of the major concerns that young people have about such topics. The writers read the literature, spoke with health experts, and incorporated their own life and professional experiences to pull together the most up-to-date information on health issues, particularly those of interest to adolescents and of concern in *Healthy People 2010.*

Throughout the alphabetical entries, the reader will find sidebars that separate fact from fiction. There are question-and-answer boxes that attempt to address the most common questions that youth ask about sensitive topics. In addition, readers will find a special feature called "Teens Speak"—case studies of teens with personal stories related to the topic in hand.

This may be one of the most important books you will ever read. Please share it with your friends, families, teachers, and classmates. Remember, you possess the power to control your future. One way to affect your course is through the acquisition of knowledge. Good luck and keep healthy.

NOTE TO LIBRARIANS

This book, along with the rest of the Truth About series serves as a wonderful resource for young researchers. It contains a variety of facts, case studies, and further readings that the reader can use to help answer questions, formulate new questions, or determine where to go to find more information. Even though the topics may be considered delicate by some, do not be afraid to ask patrons if they have questions. Feel free to direct them to the appropriate sources, but do not press them if you encounter reluctance. The best we can do as educators is to let young people know that we are there when they need us.

Mark J. Kittleson, Ph.D.
General Editor, First Edition

MENTAL HEALTH AND MENTAL DISORDERS

Most healthy people are able to handle stressful situations. Although they recognize that life can be challenging, they know it doesn't have to be overwhelming. If an individual feels overwhelmed constantly or has difficulty with stress, he or she may be suffering from depression or an anxiety disorder.

Generally, *fear* refers to feelings of dread, terror, or alarm about particular things or specific situations (such as flying or public speaking). Anxiety, on the other hand, evokes similar feelings, but there may be no specific object or situation causing those feelings, or the feeling may be out of proportion to what most people feel. Anxiety disorders refer to an emotional state characterized by feelings of intense or frequent anxiety that cause an individual difficulty or distress.

NEW IN THE REVISED EDITION

In the United States, an estimated 26.2 percent of those age 18 and older suffer from a diagnosable **mental disorder.** That means that about 57.7 million people have some type of psychological, or mental health, issue. In this new edition of *The Truth About Anxiety and Depression,* you will find updated information on the variety of problems that millions of people face each day. You also will find new entries on the genetics of mood and anxiety disorders, gender and depression, ethnicity and depression, types of psychotherapy available, mental health professionals, and related disorders.

Not all of the new information is encouraging. For example, the suicide rate in the United States is on the rise. A recent study found that from 1999 to 2005, the overall suicide rate in the United States rose 0.7 percent. In addition, researchers at Harvard Medical Center report that childhood depression is rapidly increasing at a rate of 23 percent each year. According to some studies, 10 percent of children suffer from depression that is so severe it greatly affects their lives and their ability to function.

One of the most unsettling studies outlined in this new edition focuses on the use of prescription drugs for nonmedical purposes. Specifically, teenagers are increasingly turning to the use of prescription medications to support their dependence on illegal drugs. According to one government study, as many as 15 percent of high school seniors abuse prescription drugs such as the painkillers Oxy-Contin and Vicodin. In fact, in the United States, the prescriptions written for stimulants increased from 5 million in 1991 to almost 35 million in 2007, while the number of prescriptions for Oxycontin and Vicodin increased from 40 million in 1991 to 180 million in 2007. The National Institute on Drug Abuse reports that 20 percent of the U.S. population use prescription drugs for nonmedical purposes. In 2008, the Centers for Disease Control and Prevention (CDC) reported that prescription drug abuse replaced heroin and cocaine in the major of fatal overdoses. The CDC said from 1999 to 2004, overdose deaths from prescription drugs such as Viodin and Oxycotin increased 142 percent, while fatal overdoses from heroin decreased 9 percent.

The mental health conditions discussed in this new edition do not only affect those suffering from depression. On the contrary, we all pay some price when someone gets sick. Researchers report that mental disorders cost the United States roughly $193 billion each year in lost earnings, according to a 2008 study by the National Institute of Mental Health (NIMH), published in the *American Journal of Psychiatry.* In addition to lost earnings, society incurs other costs: Some people with untreated mental disorders are also incarcerated or living on the street.

Mental disorders have a greater impact on specific minority groups than on the general population. Recent studies show that white Americans have better access to proper health treatment than such minorities as African Americans, Hispanics, and Native Americans. When it comes to race, mental health services are complex and uneven. Those who are better educated and earn more money are more likely to receive proper treatment for depression and other behavioral issues than the poor.

Although getting the right kind of help requires some research, anxiety and depression can be treated. In the new entry on types of psychotherapies, a long list of "Mental Health Treatments"—and what they do—will help anyone to get started if he or she is suffering from anxiety or depression.

DEFINING TERMS

Depression and anxiety disorders are types of mental disorders. A mental disorder is a psychological, or mental, state that has distressful, sometimes life-altering, effects ranging from sleep problems or relationship troubles to drug addiction or suicide.

Mental disorders affect people of all ages, racial and ethnic groups, and educational and socioeconomic levels.

According to the National Alliance on Mental Illness

- Twenty percent of adults in the United States, or about 40 million people, experience some type of mental disorder each year.
- Ten million U.S. adults have a serious mental illness
- Ten percent of children and adolescents suffer from mental illness severe enough to cause some level of impairment
- Those between the ages of 15 and 24 years old are more likely to experience a major bout of depression compared to other age groups
- Fifty to 60 percent of Americans with severe mental disorders also abuse drugs and alcohol, compared with 10 percent in the general population.

Theories vary about the causes of mental disorders. Mental disorders may occur after traumatic events, alongside other psychological difficulties, or for no apparent reason. Close relatives of people with mental disorders are sometimes more likely to develop the same disorder than people in other families. This phenomenon has led some researchers to report a genetic cause for mental disorders. *Genetic* is a term that refers to characteristics that are inherited, such as hair or eye color. Most mental disorders have a biological component. There are chemicals in the brain that can cause mental disorders when the chemical levels are higher or lower than normal, or if the chemicals are not properly balanced. However, for many disorders, it is not clear whether the chemical imbalance is a cause or a symptom of the disorder.

To help psychologists diagnose mental disorders, each has been named, categorized, and described. These definitions appear in a reference manual, *Diagnostic and Statistical Manual of Mental Disorders, Fourth Edition (DSM-IV)*, published in 2001 by the American Psychiatric Association. The *DSM-IV* is the set of guidelines used by mental health professionals to diagnose all mental disorders. This book discusses two mental disorders that are defined in the *DSM-IV*: depression and anxiety disorders.

Sometimes the term *depression* is used to refer to a normal human emotion, feeling sad or blue. After failing a test or breaking up with a boyfriend or girlfriend, you may tell people you're depressed. But depression is actually a long-lasting mental disorder involving deep levels of hopelessness and despair. This level of depression usually requires professional treatment.

Bipolar disorder, or manic-depressive illness, is a mental disorder that includes depression. The National Institute of Mental Health (NIMH) defines *bipolar disorder* as a brain disorder that causes unusual shifts in mood, energy, and ability to function. Bipolar disorder is a kind of depression that includes periods of **mania,** times of extreme excitement or irritability. Unlike the normal ups and downs that everyone experiences, the symptoms of bipolar disorder and depression are severe.

WHAT ARE THE SYMPTOMS AND EFFECTS OF ANXIETY AND DEPRESSION?

Although anxiety and depression are not the same, depression and anxiety disorders have similar symptoms. Both people who are depressed and those who suffer from anxiety disorders may be subject to mood swings. Both may withdraw from their usual activities. They may not be able to talk with their friends, family, coworkers, or fellow students as they did before suffering from these disorders. They may not be able to tell friends or loved ones how they are feeling, and they may even lie about how they feel in order to be left alone.

According to the National Mental Health Association (NMHA), almost half of all people diagnosed with an anxiety disorder also suffer from depression. The NMHA (2003) also reported that two out of three people diagnosed with depression exhibit symptoms of anxiety.

Despite similarities in symptoms such as social isolation, sleep problems, and loss of energy, depression and anxiety disorders are not the same. Anxiety disorders can develop without signs of depression, and people living with depression may not experience anxiety symptoms.

Symptoms of depression

Those who suffer from depression may feel hopeless, overwhelmed, or angry. Their energy level may be low, making simple day-to-day tasks seem difficult. They may not be able to maintain relationships that are important to them. They often have changes in their sleep, appetite, concentration, and memory. If their feelings of hopelessness last for a long period of time and interfere with their ability to function, they may be diagnosed with depression.

The National Institute of Mental Health (NIMH) estimates that almost 19 million American adults suffer from depression at some time during their lifetimes. NIMH also reports that women are about twice as likely as men to develop depression. Although depression can occur at any age, including the teen years, the median age of onset is 32.

Anxiety disorders

Those who suffer from an anxiety disorder experience fear, **panic,** or anxiety in situations where most people don't feel anxious or threatened. Panic is an intense feeling of fear or anxiety that comes on suddenly; the feeling may be overwhelming and seem to be unfounded. Some people experience sudden **panic attacks** without knowing what the **trigger** was. A trigger is an event, feeling, or situation that prompts a panic or anxiety attack. Other people feel constantly worried or anxious. Without treatment, such disorders can make it difficult to go to school, be with friends, or even leave one's house.

Anxiety disorders are common in the United States. According to the NIMH, more than 19 million Americans suffer from anxiety disorders.

PREVALENCE OF MENTAL DISORDERS IN TEENS

Many teens experience mental disorders that interfere with their normal development and daily lives. According to a wide-ranging study entitled "Methodology for Epidemiology of Mental Disorders in Children and Adolescents," almost 8.4 million children ages nine to 17 in the United States, or one out of five children, had a diagnosable mental or addictive disorder associated with at least minimum impairment. A total of 4.3 million children had a significant impairment at home, at school, and with peers. Sometimes teens are not diagnosed with these mental disorders because the symptoms of anxiety and depression can be similar to characteristics associated with healthy teenagers. For example, many teenagers are moody and irritable simply because of the pressures of life and the impact of adolescent hormones. These behaviors resemble the moodiness and irritability that are common symptoms in people suffering from anxiety or depression.

Some mental disorders are mild, while others are more severe. The more severe the disorder, the more likely it is to disrupt the sufferer's daily life. Some disorders persist for only short periods of time, while others can last a lifetime. According to the U.S. Surgeon General, 10 percent of children and adolescents had mental illnesses severe enough to affect their daily lives. This report also stated that the most common mental illnesses among children and adolescents are anxiety disorders. About half of those children and adolescents had a second anxiety disorder or other mental disorder, such as depression. The NIMH reports that up to 3 percent of children and up to 8 percent of teens in the United States experience depression.

Help is available. Most teens who suffer from mental disorders can lead normal lives if they receive treatment.

THE BEHAVIORS ASSOCIATED WITH MENTAL DISORDERS

Untreated mental disorders usually affect a person's ability to carry out day-to-day activities. The behaviors and symptoms of depression and anxiety disorders range from mild, such as feeling tired, to severe, such as abusing drugs or alcohol.

Signs of depression or anxiety disorders

If feelings of sadness or discouragement last more than a few weeks or take control of a person's life, those feelings may be signs of a mental disorder.

According to the *Diagnostic and Statistical Manual of Mental Disorders, Fourth Edition (DSM-IV),* people who suffer from mental disorders like depression or anxiety are likely to display one or more of the following behaviors:

■ feelings of worthlessness, hopelessness, helplessness, total indifference, and/or extreme guilt

■ prolonged sadness, unexplained crying spells

■ jumpiness or irritability

■ withdrawal from formerly enjoyable activities or relationships

■ inability to concentrate or remember details

■ loss of appetite or great increase in appetite

■ constant fatigue or insomnia

■ physical ailments that cannot be explained otherwise

■ thoughts of death or suicide attempts

If you are experiencing any of these symptoms, talk with someone about your feelings. You don't have to suffer in silence. You are not alone. There are people who can help you feel better. You can talk to a teacher, a religious counselor, a physician, or some other adult you trust. They can help you find the professional help you may need.

Common health problems
In addition to psychological or mental symptoms, both depression and anxiety disorders can wreak havoc on a person's body. The two can make existing medical conditions worse and may even increase the likelihood of some diseases, such as cancer or heart disease. Conditions associated with mental disorders include the following:

■ **Insomnia.** Many people with mental disorders have difficulty sleeping. They may have trouble falling asleep, wake up frequently during the night, or awaken in the early hours of the morning and be unable to go back to sleep. Treating mental disorders can improve sleep patterns and allow the sufferer to wake up feeling rested.

■ Weight problems. Some people who suffer from anxiety disorders or depression overeat, resulting in significant weight gain. Being overweight is associated with many health risks, including increased risk of heart disease, high blood pressure, and diabetes. Other people may be unable to eat, resulting in significant weight loss. Being too thin is also associated with many health risks.

■ Lack of energy. People who experience mental disorders, particularly depression, frequently lack energy and motivation, get little exercise, and become physically unfit. Even people who were formerly active may stop exercising. Combining exercise and a healthy diet with treatment for mental disorders can reduce risks associated with poor fitness and an unhealthy weight.

■ Heart disease, stroke, and high blood pressure. According to the Centers for Disease Control and Prevention, mental disorders are a risk factor for developing high blood pressure, a major cause of heart disease and stroke. A risk factor is a way of describing a person's increased likelihood of suffering from a mental disorder or disease.

Other physical problems that may result from anxiety or depression include ongoing physical symptoms, such as headaches, **chronic pain,** and digestive problems that do not respond to treatment. By seeking treatment for mental disorders, people feel better not only emotionally but also physically.

THE EFFECTS OF MENTAL DISORDERS

Mental disorders such as depression or anxiety disorders can affect not only the mind and body but also relationships.

Relationship difficulties

Those who suffer from mental disorders often find that they have problems with people who are close to them. Strong friendships may suddenly deteriorate and strained relationships may worsen. A person who experiences a mental disorder may do hurtful things, lash out at friends, or say things they don't mean. They may express anger with family and friends. Such behaviors can cause hurt feelings and damage relationships.

Healthy people may find it difficult to be with someone who is suffering from a mental disorder, because of unpredictable behavior and even personality changes. The person may become excessively impulsive or angry, causing problems within a family or among friends. Someone with an anxiety disorder who enjoyed going out could turn into someone who rarely leaves the house. Someone who was fun to be with may become a person who views the world as dark and hopeless.

If someone you know is behaving differently than usual, talk to an adult about it. Bearing the weight of a friend or family member's mental disorder is too much for one person. In these situations, the support of a trustworthy adult or a professional who is trained to deal with mental disorders can be beneficial.

Social consequences

Mental disorders can lead to alcohol or drug abuse, violence, or suicide. To a person with a mental disorder, life's difficulties seem much more intense.

People suffering from mental disorders are more likely to commit crimes. According to the Office of Juvenile Justice and Delinquency Prevention, each year at least one out of every five young people in the juvenile justice system has a serious mental health problem.

Substance abuse among people suffering from mental disorders is common. Substance abuse describes the excessive use of drugs or alcohol. Using alcohol and other drugs to "drown sorrows" is one way that people of all ages try to ease the pain of their symptoms. But drinking or taking drugs to ease depression or anxiety creates a vicious cycle. Drugs and alcohol alter the mental state and interfere with chemicals in the brain. Therefore they can make mental disorders more severe.

School and work performance

Mental disorders can interfere with a person's ability to succeed in school or at work. Depression and anxiety make concentration and memory difficult, which in turn affects a person's ability to carry out his or her responsibilities. A person may have trouble getting out of bed and making it to school on time, or come home from school and sleep through the afternoon shift at work.

Mood swings are common with both anxiety and depression. A person experiencing either disorder may uncharacteristically scream at an employer or teacher. Motivation to do well in school or at work often declines. The result may be failing grades or the loss of a job.

Treating mental disorders can reduce pressure at school or work by improving the person's concentration level. Treatment can also help him or her sleep better, providing more energy during the day.

EFFECTIVENESS OF TREATMENT

Sometimes people suffering from mental disorders don't receive treatment, because they don't recognize the symptoms as part of a pattern. They may blame their symptoms on the flu, lack of sleep, stress, or poor diet. If left untreated, mental disorders worsen and may even lead to death from medical complications or suicide (intentionally taking one's own life). When people recognize the symptoms and patterns of mental disorders early and seek treatment, they can avoid needless suffering and possible danger. According to the National Alliance on Mental Illness, the economic costs of untreated mental illness in the United States is more than $100 billion year. In addition, the U.S. Surgeon General reports that 80 percent of children who need mental health services do not get those services. Additionally, the Surgeon General says that 80 to 90 percent of mental disorders are treatable.

Learning about depression and anxiety disorders can help one determine if a problem exists. If someone you know has any of the symptoms of mental disorders, or if you have them, don't keep these problems to yourself. Talk to an adult you trust, such as a teacher, coach, counselor, or doctor. Identifying mental disorders early can prevent serious consequences. According to the National Institutes of Health, 77 percent of those who attempted suicide between the ages of 10 and 18 did not attend or failed to complete recommended treatment programs.

RISKY BUSINESS SELF TEST: TRUE OR FALSE?

If you are wondering whether you might be experiencing depression or an anxiety disorder, the following self-test can help you learn more about yourself. Your responses will not give you a diagnosis, but they may help you gain insight into what you are feeling. Remember, there is no substitute for the opinions and advice of a professional mental health worker.

List all statements that are true for you:

Feelings

I feel sad and irritable much of the time.

I often feel afraid to be alone.

I feel lonely most of the time.

I feel hopeless most of the time.

I seem more depressed than my friends.

Other people have noticed changes in my moods.

I have trouble concentrating and remembering things.

I have trouble making decisions.

Nothing is interesting to me.

I can't seem to get along with anyone.

I get angry all the time.

I cry all the time.

I hate myself.

Behaviors

I sometimes use alcohol, tobacco, and other drugs.

I have lost interest in activities I once enjoyed.

Other people have noticed changes in my activity level.

I avoid places I used to go that now make me feel uncomfortable.

My grades are getting worse.

I've gotten in trouble with my teachers or my boss at work.

Health and well-being

I sometimes think about suicide and ending it all.

I have made a plan to commit suicide.

I have attempted suicide.

I have had a panic attack, with a fast heartbeat, shortness of breath, and sweaty palms.

I have trouble with sleep—I sleep too much or not enough.

I have trouble with my appetite—I eat too much or not enough.

Listing any one of these items as true for you does not mean you are suffering from a mental disorder. However, if you selected more than one statement, it is probably a good idea to talk with someone about how you are feeling. If you selected more than a few statements, please talk to someone right away. The school nurse, a doctor, a teacher, or any adult you trust would be a good choice. He or she can help you find a counselor to talk to, if you wish.

If you or someone you care about has been thinking about suicide, you should speak with a professional immediately or call 911. Your feelings are important and need to be taken seriously. The United States Suicide Hotline (800-784-2433) is also available to anyone thinking about suicide.

See also: Anxiety Disorders; Anxiety Disorders, Symptoms of; Depression and Substance Abuse; Depression, Causes of; Depression, Symptoms of; Social Costs of Anxiety and Depression

A-TO-Z ENTRIES

■ ANXIETY DISORDERS

Mental disorders characterized by feelings of fear. Anxiety is a feeling similar to fear but, unlike fear, it may be a result of an imagined danger.

Everyone experiences anxiety at one time or another. When people are frightened and are not sure how to respond to a situation, they feel anxious. Anxiety becomes a mental disorder when the symptoms are so severe and long lasting that they have a negative effect on a person's life—he or she may lose sleep, have trouble at school or work, or have difficulty maintaining friendships and other relationships. Anxiety has physical symptoms such as headache, stomach upset, or perspiration.

Anxiety disorders may develop gradually over long periods of time or appear suddenly. No matter how they develop, they are relatively common psychological conditions and are treatable.

TEENS SPEAK

How I Discovered That My Feelings Were More Intense than "Normal"

The last time it happened was right before the holiday band performance. I had a solo—I play the saxophone—and I was nervous about it. The morning of the concert, I woke up at five even though I didn't need to get up until seven. I lay there, feeling paralyzed. I didn't know it then, but I was experiencing anxiety.

By seven that morning I was okay, but those two hours were awful. All I did was think about the performance and how I was going to mess it up. I saw myself standing on the stage, spotlight glaring on me, and I couldn't get a single note to come out of the sax without a really loud SQUAWK.

Later that night, just before I was ready to go on stage, I thought I was having a heart attack. It felt as if my heart was going to explode. I felt tingling in my arm, and I couldn't get a good breath of air. I felt as if I were smothering. I grabbed the curtain at the side of the stage to keep myself from falling. Our band director came over and asked if I was okay, but I couldn't answer her. I just stared at her, knowing I was going to die.

The next thing I remembered was waking up at the hospital. They tell me I had passed out. After running lots of tests and talking to many doctors, they told me I had experienced a panic attack. That's when I finally told everyone about how often this happened to me. A big test, a party, even getting lunch in the cafeteria was enough to give me what I thought was a heart attack. I always thought I was just a shy person who might have a bad heart. I never told anyone about it, because I thought that's what everyone went through.

The doctors told me that with therapy and maybe some medication, I would be just fine. I'm glad I am not dying and that I don't have to feel that way anymore.

LEARNED BEHAVIORS

Anxiety is a learned behavior. It may originate in family interactions. For example, parents may set very high standards of achievement for their child. If children interpret their parents' wishes as harsh demands, they may develop an anxiety disorder in the struggle to meet those expectations.

Other childhood incidents can also lead to unhealthy beliefs about oneself. Even small events can seem important to a sensitive person, whether he or she has a mental disorder or not. An anxiety disorder can develop as the result of frequent criticism or being put down on a regular basis. Lack of affection, encouragement, or support from family members can also increase the likelihood of experiencing an anxiety disorder.

SPECIFIC EXPERIENCES

Specific events can activate anxiety disorders, but usually only individuals who already have psychological, inherited, or physical **predispositions,** such as a certain kind of brain chemistry, are susceptible. A predisposition is a condition that makes an individual more likely to suffer from a disease. Some people may even have a predisposition to a specific fear. For example, suppose a person was once frightened by a spider. That single experience may be enough to cause a fear of spiders in the future.

Frightening experiences, such as a house fire or being bitten by a dog, can lead to anxiety in similar situations in the future. The memory of the experience can be so traumatizing that a person reacts with undue anxiety every time something similar happens, such as seeing a fire in a fireplace or encountering a friendly dog.

PSYCHOLOGICAL FACTORS

Anxiety is not always caused by an event. More often than not, **self-talk** stirs up anxiety and makes it stronger. Self-talk is what people say to themselves when everyday stresses occur. Negative self-talk can intensify anxiety. Even if a biological reason prompted the anxiety initially, self-talk can keep it growing. By the time people have finished scaring themselves, their anxiety has probably lasted longer than it would have without the negative commentary. For example, if you were invited to a party but didn't want to go, you might use negative self-talk to convince yourself you will lose all your friends if you say no. You can create a situation that is filled with anxiety simply by what you say to yourself. Those who learn to deal effectively with stressful situations are less likely to turn symptoms of anxiety into full-fledged anxiety disorders.

PHYSIOLOGICAL FACTORS

Anxiety has physical and biological causes. Your body is designed to respond to threats. This natural response is often called the **fight-or-flight** response. It originates in the brain, especially the region of the lower brain called the locus ceruleus, which controls emotional responses. During this automatic, involuntary response, the brain releases increased quantities of chemicals that cause the adrenal glands to release more **adrenaline.**

Adrenaline is a chemical that speeds up your heartbeat and breathing. Your body starts sending blood to your most vital areas and restricts blood flow to extremities and other less important areas of the body. Blood sugar, lactic acid, and other chemicals are also released. All of these responses prepare the body to fight or flee from a perceived danger (such as a house fire or a mugger). Common feelings include dread, fear, and a sense of impending doom.

Many anxiety disorders can lead to **panic attacks**—episodes of extreme anxiety that can include heavy perspiration, feelings of suffocation, and a rapid heart rate. Scientists have discovered that these symptoms result from the stimulation of a particular region of the brain

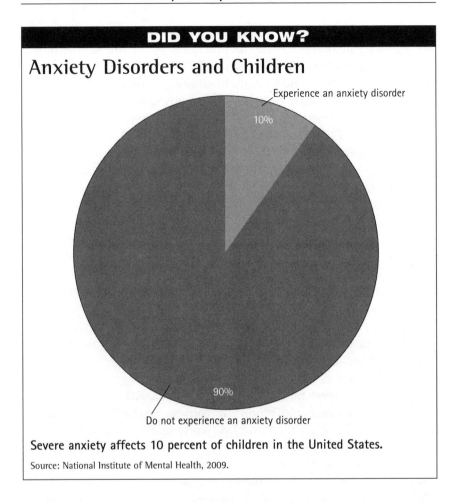

DID YOU KNOW?

Anxiety Disorders and Children

Experience an anxiety disorder

10%

90%

Do not experience an anxiety disorder

Severe anxiety affects 10 percent of children in the United States.

Source: National Institute of Mental Health, 2009.

that sets off a fight-or-flight response. A panic attack can be disrupted with medication or by slightly damaging the locus ceruleus in the brain.

Some anxiety symptoms are the result of an insufficient amount of gamma aminobutyric acid (GABA), a chemical that calms the brain. GABA actually works by suppressing the normal fight-or-flight alarm. Those who have enough GABA stay calm; those who do not have enough can develop anxiety symptoms.

Certain medical conditions can also cause symptoms of anxiety and panic. In fact, more than 50 physical conditions—including **diabetes** and **hypoglycemia**—may cause anxiety. Diabetes is a disorder in which the body is not able to control its levels of blood sugar. Diabetes can cause kidney, eye, and nerve damage. Hypoglycemia is also related to the body's ability to regulate sugar. It occurs when the body does not produce enough sugar. Inner ear disturbances may cause anxiety symptoms to develop as well.

A relatively harmless heart condition called **mitral valve prolapse** may also act as a **trigger** for a panic attack. Those who have the condition have a valve in their heart—the mitral valve—that does not close fully after blood has passed from one chamber to another. They may feel an extra heartbeat or a stronger beat than usual. The symptom usually goes away with no harm done. However, some individuals interpret these erratic heartbeats as the beginning of a panic attack or heart attack. If they react with alarm, their anxiety level increases, and they may indeed suffer a panic attack (although they will not experience a heart attack). According to the Substance Abuse and Mental Health Services Administration, about 10 of every 100 children experience anxiety disorders.

DRUG USE

Artificially stimulating the body with chemicals can also cause anxiety. The National Institute of Mental Health (NIMH) reported in 2001 that stimulants—drugs such as caffeine, nicotine, amphetamines, and cocaine—provoke anxiety reactions. Stimulants are often referred to as "uppers." These drugs tend to increase alertness, energy, and physical activity. They produce what is often called a "rush," by stimulating the nervous system. The NIMH also reports that caffeine alone might cause panic attacks. Anxiety is also likely to occur as people withdraw from drug use, including alcohol.

ENVIRONMENT

Certain environmental toxins (such as insecticides, mercury, and lead) can cause anxiety. These toxins affect the brain and can activate the fight-or-flight response that may lead to a panic attack.

Threats to safety, the death of a loved one, the breakup of a relationship, difficulties at home, or failing grades can all cause high levels of anxiety or even an anxiety disorder in the short term. Major life changes, such as moving to a new city, changing jobs, having children, or starting a new relationship can trigger high levels of anxiety and panic attacks as well.

See also: Anxiety Disorders, Common Types of; Anxiety Disorders, Symptoms of; Related Disorders

FURTHER READING
Bourne, Edmund J. *The Anxiety & Phobia Workbook.* 4th ed. Oakland, Calif.: New Harbinger Publications, 2005.

■ ANXIETY DISORDERS, COMMON TYPES OF

Mental disorders causing biological changes in the brain as a result of fears that are out of control. The most common anxiety disorders include generalized anxiety disorder (GAD), panic disorder, agoraphobia, obsessive-compulsive disorder (OCD), phobias, and post-traumatic stress disorder (PTSD).

Anxiety disorders are the most common form of mental illness in the United States. They affect 40 million adults, or 18.1 percent of the adult population (ages 18–54), according to the Anxiety Disorders Association of America. Anxiety disorders are also the most common mental health problems for children and teens. The Substance Abuse and Mental Health Services Administration reports that 10 percent of children have an anxiety disorder.

Q & A

Question: I was recently diagnosed with depression, but I keep having panic attacks—could I also have an anxiety disorder?

Answer: Yes. It is common for an anxiety disorder to accompany other mental disorders including depression, eating disorders, substance abuse, or even another anxiety disorder. Anxiety disorders can also happen if you are suffering from a physical illness such as cancer or heart disease. If you are being treated for one mental or physical disorder but continue to have symptoms that are troubling, be sure to talk to your doctor or therapist about the symptoms.

GENERALIZED ANXIETY DISORDER

Generalized Anxiety Disorder (GAD) is a condition characterized by a long period of excessive worry and anxiety that is difficult to control. People can be diagnosed with GAD if these symptoms persist for six or more months. People with GAD tend to worry constantly about academic performance, sporting activities, social relationships, or work, even when there are no signs of trouble. Sometimes they aren't worried about anything in particular but feel tense and stressed all day long. They may also have physical symptoms such as low energy, chest pains, muscle tension, headaches, or irritability. Everyone worries sometimes, but those who have GAD stay worried. They fear that the absolute worst will happen and rarely are able to relax.

According to the Anxiety Disorders Association of America GAD affects about 6.8 million of Americans in the course of their lives and is more common in women than in men. GAD usually begins in childhood and can become a serious problem if left untreated. Some experts believe that it is underdiagnosed and more common than other anxiety disorders.

GAD usually first appears in childhood or the teenage years. Typically, it occurs in tense young people who need more reassurance about their appearance, intelligence, or social acceptance than most people do. They are usually eager to please others and may be **perfectionists**—never satisfied with their own less-than-perfect performance. Like most anxiety disorders, GAD can be successfully treated with medicine and therapy.

TEENS SPEAK

I Lived with
Obsessive-Compulsive Disorder

My obsessive-compulsive disorder (OCD) started when I was about nine. I used to worry constantly that something bad would happen to my mom and the worries would disturb my whole day.

As I got older, the worries got worse. When I went to the cafeteria, I would feel totally overwhelmed because I had to decide what to eat. I was always afraid of making a mistake. I never wanted to make the wrong choice and it affected my performance at school, my friendships—everything. I just couldn't make decisions because I didn't trust myself.

Before I began treatment for OCD, I was afraid of touching anything, and I mean anything! I would wash my hands hundreds of times a day. My hands would get red and raw from all the scrubbing, but when I put on moisturizer they'd feel dirty again. I'd have to sit touching nothing, with my hands up my sleeves, to "protect" myself.

And it wasn't just being afraid of getting dirty. My obsessive thoughts made me chronically late for everything. I was late for school all the time. Sometimes I couldn't get out of the house because I would check myself over and over, wondering "Did I do this?" or "Did I do that?" It made me miss school, and I definitely failed at least one class because of it.

I didn't think there was any hope, but I was desperate, afraid I'd fail out of school and have no friends. It was getting harder and harder to hide my OCD symptoms. I talked to a teacher who was especially nice to me and she gave me the phone number of a therapist who specialized in treating anxiety disorders like OCD. I talked to my therapist and she prescribed medication to help me with the disease.

After a couple of months of therapy and medication, my symptoms were under control. Thank goodness, my doubts and obsessions are now manageable. I know there are people out there who have OCD and don't know what it is. You aren't crazy! Just talk to someone about it, a mental health professional, and be honest with them. It can get better; it did for me!

PANIC DISORDER, OR "PANIC ATTACKS"

Panic is the body's healthy way of preparing you to fight or run away when encountering a threat. A **panic attack** is a period of extreme anxiety with physical symptoms such as heart palpitations, shakiness, dizziness, and racing thoughts. A panic attack can occur in combination with other anxiety disorders. For example, people with phobias or obsessive-compulsive disorder may experience panic attacks as symptoms of their disorder. According to the NIMH, a panic disorder is "characterized by unexpected and repeated" panic attacks. The number and severity of the attacks varies widely among those with a panic disorder, but the concern about having further attacks and changing behavior to avoid such attacks are the key characteristics.

The National Mental Health Association (NMHA) reported in 2004 that more than 2.4 million Americans suffer from panic attacks annually. The NMHA also revealed that panic disorders typically appear in young adulthood. In fact, about half of all people who have panic disorder developed the condition before age 24.

Physiology of panic attacks

A panic attack causes two parts of the nervous system to react to protect you and your body: the **sympathetic nervous system (SNS)** and the **parasympathetic nervous system (PNS).** The job of the SNS is to stir or energize and the job of the PNS is to restore calm. The two parts balance each other.

When you are frightened, the SNS releases adrenaline and your heart pumps harder to make your blood circulate more quickly to the places it is most needed. You're only aware of your pounding, racing heart or tingling sensations in your hands and feet. Your lungs work harder to draw in more air. You start to breathe harder and faster. You begin to sweat. The adrenaline causes you to focus more intensely on the immediate danger. Your body is now totally immersed in the **fight-or-flight response.**

Were it not for the PNS, your body would suffer because it would be constantly ready to fight (or run). So, once the danger has passed, the PNS takes over, stopping the flow of adrenaline and returning your body to a relaxed state.

A panic attack occurs when the body has heightened responses even though there is no immediate danger. The body isn't required to react, because there is no threat. Therefore it has no way of getting rid of the adrenaline. Eventually, the PNS kicks in and the symptoms diminish. In the meantime, you may be left feeling frighteningly intense symptoms. Since you see no visible danger, you may decide the threat is within your own body. You may think you're having a heart attack when it is actually a panic attack.

Facts about panic attacks

- Panic attacks often begin during teenage years and early adulthood. The NMHA (2004) reported that roughly half of all people who have panic disorder develop the condition before age 24.
- A typical panic attack lasts for two to 10 minutes but can even last up to an hour.
- The aftereffects of a panic attack—anxiety—can linger for hours or even days.
- In the United States, 1.7 percent of the adult population, or 2.4 million people, have a panic disorder in a given year, according to a 2004 report by the NMHA.
- The NMHA also notes that women are affected twice as frequently as men.

PHOBIA

A phobia is a persistent, irrational fear of an object, activity, or situation. Fear is a normal response to danger. It can be helpful in preparing to escape from or confront a threat. Because fear causes the heart and the lungs to work faster, you are better able to fight or flee, whichever makes sense under the circumstances.

Fear becomes a phobia only when a person alters his or her lifestyle in order to manage that fear. A phobia is a fear that is out of control—far beyond what is reasonable under the circumstances. The fear is no longer an aid to survival and it can hinder leading a normal, healthy life.

There are two general categories of phobia: specific and social. When people are afraid of particular things, they are said to be suffering from **specific phobia**. Objects or situations that may act as a **trigger** for phobia include contact with snakes or insects, being in a storm or an airplane, or being on a bridge or in a small space.

Social phobia is marked by a persistent fear of being in a situation where one may be embarrassed. For example, a person with social phobia might imagine standing in front of a room full of classmates and suddenly discovering an obvious stain on his or her shirt. A person with social phobia might panic at the idea of eating in a restaurant for fear of spilling food or stumbling into a table. If the phobic condition is severe enough, the situation may set off a panic attack.

The fear of social situations experienced by those with a social phobia is not simply a result of low self-esteem. Increasing one's self-confidence does not rid a person of a social phobia. He or she is also unlikely to "grow out of it." The fears associated with social phobia are irrational and uncontrollable, but knowing they are irrational does not make them go away. In fact, the inability to get rid of the fears may lead to low self-esteem. Some people who suffer from the disorder may be overly critical of themselves if they are unable to rid themselves of fears they know are unwarranted.

A social phobia can be thought of as a false alarm. Despite logic and even a recognition that a situation isn't dangerous or life-threatening, the body reacts as if there is a serious threat and prepares for a fight or flight. Recent research indicates that specific chemical systems in the brain may be responsible for the signs and symptoms of social phobia.

Fact Or Fiction?

Anxiety disorders are best treated by simply "pulling oneself together" or by "talking things out" with someone.

The Facts: Anxiety disorders are best treated by a professional health-care provider using medication, specific therapy techniques, or a combination of the two.

Fear of social situations cannot be treated by simply talking with a friend. In fact, because people with social phobias know their anxiety is out of proportion to what the situation deserves, talking rationally does little to help. The best way to treat a social phobia is with the medication and specific therapy techniques that only a health-care professional can offer. Medications used for social phobia include certain kinds of antidepressants (even though the person may not suffer from depression). Therapy techniques for phobias include relaxation techniques and programs for gradual exposure to feared situations. The most beneficial treatments often combine medication with psychotherapy.

AGORAPHOBIA

Agoraphobia literally means "a fear of the marketplace." Those who suffer from agoraphobia experience severe anxiety about being in open spaces or public areas. They may fear grocery stores, malls, other people's houses, or school—just about any place except the safety of their own home.

Typically, the sufferer fears panic symptoms in a place where escape may prove either difficult or embarrassing. Agoraphobia can keep sufferers from ordinary responsibilities and tasks such as going to school or work, doing the grocery shopping, or visiting a doctor.

OBSESSIVE-COMPULSIVE DISORDER

An obsessive-compulsive disorder (OCD) is characterized by distressing thoughts that don't go away, and repeating certain behaviors (like washing one's hands or touching certain objects) or mental acts (like praying or counting) to cancel out those thoughts. OCD is a serious disorder. In 2009, the World Health Organization ranked obsessive-compulsive disorder as one of the top 10 disabilities in the world.

An obsessive-compulsive disorder has two distinct parts: **obsessions** and **compulsions**. Obsessions are thoughts that won't go away. They are unwanted, uncontrollable, and often inappropriate, such as the thought of intentionally crashing a car into a brick wall. Compulsions develop in response to obsessions. Being driven—or compelled—to repeat certain physical or mental tasks over and over helps people with OCD find relief from the anxiety of the obsession.

Everyone has inappropriate thoughts from time to time and everyone has routines. If a routine or recurring thought interferes with one's life, however, he or she may be suffering from an obsessive-compulsive disorder.

The most common obsessions concern thoughts of contamination. Some people suffering from OCD worry about contact with dirt or germs from almost any source. They may fear shaking hands, eating, and even opening doors.

The most common compulsion is called **checking**. Checking means repeatedly inspecting or revisiting something one has done to see if it was actually done. Some people have to keep checking to see if they locked the front door, brought in the newspaper, or turned out the lights. They don't just check once or twice; they may check 20 or 30 times.

POST-TRAUMATIC STRESS DISORDER

Post-traumatic stress disorder, or PTSD, is a mental disorder that affects individuals who have experienced or witnessed life-threatening events such as sexual, physical, or emotional abuse, military combat, natural disasters, a terrorist action, a serious accident, or a violent assault like rape.

People who suffer from PTSD often relive the experience through nightmares and flashbacks. Flashbacks are memories of previous experiences that are vivid, realistic, and often frightening. PTSD sufferers also may have difficulty sleeping. They often feel detached from other people as well. These symptoms can be severe enough and last long enough to significantly affect a person's daily life. The symptoms may appear immediately after the traumatic event or events or many years later. It may take people with PTSD months or years—even with professional help—before they recognize that their symptoms are related to something that happened years ago. Diagnosing PTSD is complicated by the fact that it frequently occurs alongside related disorders such as depression, substance abuse, or memory problems. The disorder is also associated with difficulties in functioning in social or family life.

THE REALITY OF ANXIETY DISORDERS

Everyone gets nervous at times, and there are many reasonable reasons for fear in life. Your palms may sweat when you speak in front of the class. You may feel uneasy when you walk down a dark street alone at night. If you find yourself altering your life, however, or suffering serious symptoms—avoiding places, people, or things; changing your plans or daily routines because of your fears; feeling that you can't breathe or are having a heart attack—you may be experiencing an anxiety disorder. Anxiety disorders are treatable. Check out the hotline section of this book (page 177) for resources that can help.

See also: Anxiety Disorders; Anxiety Disorders, Symptoms of; Post-Traumatic Stress Disorder; Related Disorders

FURTHER READING

Anxiety Disorders—A Medical Dictionary, Bibliography, and Annotated Research Guide to Internet References. San Diego, Calif.: Icon Health Publications, 2003.

Barlow, David H. *The Nature and Treatment of Anxiety and Panic.* New York: Guilford Press, 2002.

Caldwell, Paul. *Anxiety Disorders: Everything You Need to Know.* Your Personal Health. Buffalo, N.Y.: Firefly Books, 2005.

■ ANXIETY DISORDERS, SYMPTOMS OF

Outward signs of mental disorders in the brain as a result of fears that are out of control. Anxiety disorders cause psychological and physical changes in the body in anticipation of real or imagined dangers. Those changes are symptoms or signs of an anxiety disorder. Under normal circumstances, the **fight-or-flight response** causes changes that help people cope with a threat. People with anxiety disorders experience those physical and psychological changes even when there is no danger.

Doctors may have difficulty diagnosing an anxiety disorder, because its symptoms often resemble those of other mental disorders, such as depression, or certain physical ailments. Some people may simply have nervous personalities. Doctors also cannot determine the cause of a symptom if they don't know the individual has it. If you believe you are suffering from anxiety, tell your medical doctor or find a therapist who has experience counseling people with anxiety.

PHYSICAL REACTIONS

The body's reaction to fear is to pump **adrenaline** into the bloodstream. Adrenaline is a **hormone**—a chemical substance secreted in this case by the adrenal gland and carried in the bloodstream to affect another part of the body. When adrenaline enters your bloodstream, you may feel your heart pounding (palpitations), begin to perspire, and breathe more rapidly. Your muscles may become tense and painful. You may become so weak that you faint. Your **gastrointestinal system,** which includes your stomach and digestive tract, may respond to the fear or anxiety by speeding up or slowing down (nausea, constipation, or diarrhea).

Anxiety disorders keep the body in the fight-or-flight mode. Dr. Mark J. Berber, a lecturer in psychiatry at the University of Toronto, reported in 2003 that, among other harmful effects, the constant release of adrenaline and other hormones can have a negative impact on the heart and the immune systems.

An already anxious person can easily interpret these symptoms as proof of a serious illness, increasing his or her anxiety. Reactions to fear are normal adjustments that prepare the body for conflict or escape (the fight-or-flight response).

The physical symptoms of anxiety disorders generally include headaches, gastrointestinal troubles, problems with one's immune system, dizziness, chest pain, and discomfort in other parts of the body. Another common symptom is **bruxism,** the clenching or grinding of teeth. The National Institute of Mental Health (2001) reported that medical doctors often treat these and other symptoms of anxiety without recognizing the underlying cause is an anxiety disorder.

Fact Or Fiction?

If I suffer from an anxiety disorder it's because I've done something wrong or because I'm too insecure to handle things like other people.

The Facts: Anxiety disorders are illnesses caused by a combination of biological and environmental factors. A negative self-image may actually be the result of an anxiety disorder.

EMOTIONAL REACTIONS

Fear can make you feel numb, overwhelmed, sad, or vulnerable. Other emotional symptoms include feelings of agitation, hopelessness, or irritability. You may not be able to stop worrying, even though you may realize your anxiety is more intense than it needs to be.

Anxiety can make it difficult to make decisions or concentrate. Sufferers often have a hard time trusting their own perceptions. For example, someone with an anxiety disorder may doubt physical symptoms of an illness because they are so used to "thinking themselves sick." They may need outward evidence, such as a raised temperature, before they accept that they are ill.

Anxiety disorders also hamper clear thinking. Sometimes people become hyperalert or especially vigilant, trying to prepare for whatever might happen through obsessive thoughts and worries—as if thinking about something enough can make it easier to deal with. Because anxiety disorders flood the mind with chemical activity, confusion, forgetfulness, and intrusive images and thoughts are likely to increase.

Anxiety is sometimes a result of stress. **Stress** refers to the emotional strain or discomfort that result from the pressures of life. The way you think about the stress you feel can make you more anxious. For instance, if you fear that you may have a stomach ailment, thinking obsessively about the possibility may actually bring on the sickness. You might also become very sensitive emotionally, feeling criticized, edgy, irritable, or jittery as you fret about the possibility of getting sick.

Anxiety can also make you feel confused and scared. This, too, comes from self-talk. If you tell yourself you can't cope, or are going to fail, you may start avoiding situations, fidgeting, shouting, stuttering, or crying. You may even become aggressive or have trouble relaxing. You may be startled or become upset more easily than other people, and you may have trouble sleeping.

WHAT TO DO WHEN SUFFERING FROM ANXIETY

- When you feel anxious or panicked, breathe calmly and deeply at normal, regular intervals. An occasional slow deep breath can help you relax and prevent symptoms of panic. You should avoid rapid short breaths.
- Don't fight your symptoms of anxiety by trying to wish the feelings away. Willpower is not a solution.
- Don't dwell on how it might get worse. Negativity can result in panic.
- Participate in simple, fun, interesting, and safe activities.
- Notice that when you eventually stop thinking frightening thoughts, your symptoms tend to fade.
- Humor and laughter are good ways to reduce and prevent symptoms of anxiety and panic.
- Avoid drugs (including alcohol) that are not approved by your physician. Some symptoms of anxiety and panic are associated with drugs, even over-the-counter medications.
- Maintain regular physical activity. Physical activity can be an effective way to relieve symptoms and build strength to relieve stress.
- Talk to a mental health professional if you experience symptoms of anxiety and panic that are recurrent, are severe, or seem unusual.

ANXIETY IS TREATABLE

The body's normal reaction to fear is called the fight-or-flight response. The body responds automatically to a threat by releasing chemicals such as adrenaline into the bloodstream. Those chemicals cause a series of dramatic physical changes in preparation for fight

DID YOU KNOW?

Anxiety Hurts

Almost half (47 percent) of those who suffer from an anxiety disorder report physical symptoms that disrupt their family life/home responsibilities.

Source: Freedom from Fear, 2003.

or flight. Those with anxiety disorders experience the symptoms of a fight-or-flight response even when there is no danger. Those symptoms include dry mouth, heavy breathing, an increased heart rate, and even feelings of suffocation. The symptoms of anxiety disorders are treatable when professional help is sought.

See also: Anxiety Disorders; Anxiety Disorders, Common Types of

FURTHER READING
Bourne, Edmund J. *The Anxiety & Phobia Workbook.* 4th ed. Oakland, Calif.: New Harbinger Publications, 2005.
Davidson Jonathan. *The Anxiety Book.* New York: Riverhead, 2004.
Essau, Cecilia, and Franz Petermann, eds. *Anxiety Disorders in Children and Adolescents: Epidemiology, Risk Factors and Treatment.* Vol. 4, *Biobehavioural Perspectives on Health and Disease Prevention.* New York: Brunner-Routledge, 2003.

■ BIPOLAR DISORDER

A mental disorder that causes unusual shifts in mood, energy, and ability to function, also known as manic-depressive disorder. Everyone experiences mood swings—one minute feeling great and the next feeling upset. These are normal reactions to life. Unlike most people, however, those who have bipolar disorder experience severe emotional swings. For people who have bipolar disorder, "highs" are periods of **mania,** or manic episodes, and "lows" are periods of depression, or depressive episodes. These swings can be severe, ranging from extreme energy to deep despair. The symptoms are so intense they can result in troubled relationships, poor job or school performance, and even suicide. Like diabetes or heart disease, bipolar disorder is a long-term illness that must be carefully managed by a medical professional throughout a person's life. It almost always can be treated, and people with this illness can lead full and productive lives.

TYPES AND SYMPTOMS

Between manic or depressive episodes, most people with bipolar disorder are free of symptoms, but the National Institute of Mental Health (NIMH) reports that as many as one-third of sufferers always have some symptoms.

A manic episode is diagnosed if an elevated mood occurs with three or more of the following symptoms most of the day, nearly every day, or for one week or longer. If the mood is irritable, four additional symptoms must be present. According to the NIMH, the signs and symptoms of mania include

- increased energy, activity, and restlessness
- excessively "high," exaggerated good mood
- extreme irritability
- racing thoughts and talking very fast, jumping from one idea to another
- distractibility, can't concentrate well
- little sleep needed
- unrealistic beliefs in one's abilities and powers
- poor judgment
- spending sprees
- a lasting period of behavior that is different from usual
- increased sexual drive
- abuse of drugs, particularly cocaine, alcohol, and sleeping medications
- provocative, intrusive, or aggressive behavior
- denial that anything is wrong

A depressive episode is diagnosed if five or more of the following symptoms last most of the day, nearly every day, for a period of two weeks or longer. Those signs and symptoms may include:

- lasting sad, anxious, or empty mood
- feelings of hopelessness or pessimism
- feelings of guilt, worthlessness, or helplessness
- loss of interest or pleasure in activities once enjoyed
- decreased energy, a feeling of fatigue or of being "slowed down"
- difficulty concentrating, remembering, making decisions
- restlessness or irritability
- sleeping too much, or can't sleep
- change in appetite and/or unintended weight loss or gain
- chronic pain or other persistent bodily symptoms that are not caused by physical illness or injury
- thoughts of death or suicide, or suicide attempts

Patterns and severity of symptoms, or episodes, of highs and lows, determine the various types of bipolar disorder

Bipolar I

Bipolar I, the most severe form of the illness, is marked by extreme manic episodes. In fact, episodes of mania in bipolar I may be so severe that they include symptoms of **psychosis,** or psychotic symptoms. Common psychotic symptoms are hallucinations (hearing, seeing, or otherwise sensing things not actually there) and delusions (false, strongly held but illogical beliefs). Psychotic symptoms tend to reflect the individual's extreme mood state at the time. For example, delusions of grandiosity, such as believing one is the president or has special powers or wealth, may occur during mania; delusions of guilt or worthlessness, such as believing that one is ruined and penniless or has committed some terrible crime, may appear during depression. People with bipolar disorder who have these symptoms are sometimes incorrectly diagnosed as having schizophrenia, a severe mental disorder resulting in a separation between thought processes and emotion, sometimes accompanied by delusions and erratic behavior.

In some people, symptoms of mania and depression may occur together in what is called a mixed bipolar state. Symptoms of a mixed state often include agitation, trouble sleeping, significant changes in appetite, psychosis, and suicidal thinking. A person may have a very sad, hopeless mood while at the same time feeling extremely energized.

Bipolar II

A person with bipolar II experiences hypomanic episodes rather than manic episodes. The difference between mania and **hypomania** is a matter of severity—hypomania generally does not impair daily functioning or result in hospitalization. Hypomania may feel good to the person who experiences it. Someone experiencing hypomania may perform better at school or work than he or she usually does. Without proper treatment, however, hypomania can become a severe manic episode or can turn into depression.

Cyclothymic disorder

A cyclothymic disorder is characterized by fluctuating moods involving periods of hypomania and depression. The periods of both depressive and hypomanic symptoms are shorter, less severe, and do not occur with as much regularity as experienced by those who have bipolar II or I. However, these mood swings can impair social interactions and work relationships. Many, but not all, people with cyclothymia develop a more severe form of bipolar illness.

There is also a form of the illness called bipolar disorder not otherwise specified (NOS) that does not fit into one of the above definitions.

RATES

According to the NIMH (2009), more than 2.6 million American adults, or 5.7 million Americans, have bipolar disorder. The disorder typically develops in late adolescence or early adulthood. However, some people have their first symptoms during childhood, and some develop them late in life. Bipolar disorder is often not recognized as an illness, and people may suffer for years before it is properly diagnosed and treated.

The Depression and Bipolar Support Alliance (DBSA) reported in 2004 that up to one-third of the 3.4 million children and adolescents with depression in the United States may actually be experiencing the early onset of bipolar disorder. According to the NIMH (2000), the illness may be at least as common among young people as among adults. In this study, 1 percent of adolescents ages 14 to 18 were found to have met criteria for bipolar disorder in their lifetime.

Bipolar disorder is more likely to affect children of parents who have the disorder. When one parent has bipolar disorder, the risk to each child is estimated to be 15–30 percent (DBSA, 2004). When both parents have bipolar disorder, the risk increases to 50–75 percent.

The Child and Adolescent Bipolar Foundation (CABF) reported in 2002 that until recently, a diagnosis of bipolar disorder was rarely made in childhood. The disorder can be difficult to recognize and diagnose in young people because it does not precisely fit the symptom criteria established for adults, and because its symptoms can resemble or co-occur with those of other common childhood-onset mental disorders.

The DBSA reported (2004) a significant number of children may be diagnosed in the United States with attention-deficit hyperactivity disorder (ADHD) but actually have early-onset bipolar disorder instead of, or along with, ADHD. In addition, symptoms of bipolar disorder may be mistaken for normal emotions and behaviors of children and adolescents. However, unlike normal mood changes, bipolar disorder significantly disturbs functioning in school, with friends, and at home with family.

SUICIDE

Some people with bipolar disorder become suicidal. Anyone who is thinking about committing suicide needs immediate attention, preferably from a mental health professional or a physician. Anyone who talks about suicide should be taken seriously. Risk for suicide appears to be higher earlier in the course of the illness. Therefore, recognizing bipolar disorder early and learning how best to manage it may decrease the risk of death by suicide.

If you are feeling suicidal or know someone who is:

- Call a doctor, emergency room, or 911 right away to get immediate help.
- Make sure you, or the suicidal person, are not left alone.
- Make sure that access is prevented to large amounts of medication, weapons, or other items that could be used for self-harm.

It is important to understand that suicidal feelings and actions are symptoms of an illness that can be treated. With proper treatment, suicidal feelings can be overcome.

TREATMENT

A NIMH report (2001) states that even people with severe forms of bipolar disorder can find relief with proper long-term treatment. This usually includes medication and therapy.

Doctors often prescribe "mood stabilizer" medications to help control bipolar disorder. Several different mood stabilizers are available for prescription use. People take most of these medications for years as a part of their treatment. Other medications may be added to help during the short term, when people with the disease experience brief episodes of mania or depression and need additional help.

In most cases, people with bipolar disorder can control the symptoms much more effectively with continuous treatment than on-and -off treatment. However, bipolar disorder is a serious illness even during continuous, long-term treatment. Extreme mood changes may occur at any time. To make sure treatment is as effective as it can be, people with bipolar disorder need to work closely with their doctors and communicate openly about their treatment concerns and options.

See also: Depression, Symptoms of; Suicide and Depression

FURTHER READING

"Bipolar Disorder." TeensHealth, Kidshealth.org. Available online. URL: http://kidshealth.org/teen/your_mind/mental_health/bipolar. html. Accessed March 24, 2010.

Findling, R. L, et al. *Pediatric Bipolar Disorder: A Handbook for Clinicians.* London: Martin Dunitz, Ltd., 2003.

■ CODEPENDENCY

A set of behaviors that frequently develop between family members and a person within the family who has a mental disorder. When someone in a family suffers from a mental disorder such as depression, addiction, or an anxiety disorder, everyone in the family is affected. The person who is codependent may come to believe that without his or her help the family member suffering from the disorder will fall apart.

Sometimes, family members fall into patterns of codependency around a loved one with a mental disorder.

These family members have good intentions. They want to do something to help their loved one, but they may confuse their need to be needed with their loved one's real needs.

Fact Or Fiction?

My father was diagnosed with depression. If I get good grades, come home from school early, treat my sister better, and do my chores every day, my dad will get better.

The Facts: Depression is a mental disorder that involves a chemical imbalance in the brain. While the environment around your dad can have some effect on his mood, it cannot make him happy or heal his depression. His mood will improve as his depression is treated with therapy and, possibly, medication.

Those who suffer from depression or an anxiety disorder are not responsible for every bad thing that happens to their family. However, they are responsible for their own behavior, and their behavior can affect the entire family. The person suffering from the disorder may behave in hurtful ways by lashing out verbally or withdrawing emotionally.

Watching a loved one suffer and undergo personality changes is difficult. In response, family members want to do whatever they can to help. To come to the aid of their loved one, they may develop patterns of behavior that seem helpful but ultimately hurt the person with the disorder in the long run. This kind of codependent behavior is sometimes called **enabling**, because it allows the individual with the disorder to continue without getting professional help.

TEENS SPEAK

My Father Wouldn't Get Out of Bed

I stopped having friends over because I never knew if my father would be in bed or passed out on the couch in the living room. He always wore the same dingy pajamas and never washed them. His hair was all tangled and knotted in a big mess. He stared blankly and the sour smell of booze was always around him. If I even tried to ask him to clean himself up so I could bring friends over, he'd yell at me or cry. I couldn't stand the crying.

Dad didn't open the mail anymore. I did the best I could to keep things going. I knew where his checkbook was and I was able to pay the bills for a while. But soon, the checks came back in the mail marked "insufficient funds."

I was tired. I had homework, and my after-school job, and I had to make sure my little brother had breakfast, lunch, and dinner. It was no life for a 16-year-old.

We got a call from the electric company and the man said if they didn't get paid, they would shut off our power at the end of the month. I didn't know what to do. I knew if I asked my dad, he'd break down again.

Finally, I called my grandmother. I told her what was happening. She lived in Florida, but Grandma said she and Grandpa would be at our apartment the next day.

When grandma and grandpa arrived, they talked to me and told me it wasn't my job to be the parent. They told me I had done well and that it was nice to want to be of help, but my job was to take care of my own life. I told them that it would all fall apart if I didn't do everything.

Later that night, Grandpa took me to a support group meeting. It was especially for teenagers who have parents who are sick. I had no idea other people felt the way I did, or did the crazy things I did to try and take care of their sick parents. What a relief to find out I didn't have to do that anymore!

WHAT IS CODEPENDENCY?

Codependency has been described as an addiction, a disease, learned behaviors, a psychological condition, and a personality disorder. Until recently, many dictionaries did not include the term. It has become widely used only within the past few decades to define the behaviors of spouses, children, or other family members who have a loved one who is chemically dependent or otherwise dysfunctional. More generally, the term is applied to individuals who neglect their own needs by focusing almost exclusively on the needs and behaviors of someone suffering from a mental disorder or other illness.

DIAGNOSIS

Codependency is so broadly defined that it can be difficult to diagnose. In fact, the *Diagnostic and Statistical Manual of Mental Disorders, Fourth Edition (DSM-IV),* published by the American Psychiatric Association (2000)—the main diagnostic reference used by mental health professionals in the United States—does not have a codependency category. However, the characteristics of codependency have been the subject of many books and articles.

People who are codependent often have low **self-esteem.** Some are so obsessed with other people's needs that they have trouble focusing on their own. Others behave in controlling ways and may find it difficult to show trust. They feel compelled to get involved even if their loved one does not want their assistance.

If you think you may be codependent, ask yourself the following questions based on a list prepared by Codependent Anonymous (CoDA) called "Patterns and Characteristics of CoDependency." Do you

- have trouble saying no?
- have trouble asking for help?
- adjust your behavior and conversation around getting attention and approval from others?
- feel inferior to others?
- feel that others have high expectations for you?
- become angry or irritated when you don't meet other people's expectations?
- focus a lot of mental time and attention on other people?
- have difficulty maintaining a stable relationship with a boyfriend or girlfriend?

And are you

- in and out of highly volatile (big ups and downs) relationships?
- uncomfortable when not in a relationship?
- frequently depressed?
- answering these questions with someone else's possible answers in mind?

If you answered "yes" to more than a few questions, you may be exhibiting some characteristics of codependency. For more information, see the Hotline and Help Sites section of this book.

SUBSTANCE ABUSE

The best-known examples of codependency involve families of alcoholics or addicts. Family members are often drawn into the addict's behavior. For example, they may make excuses when he or she doesn't show up for an appointment or bail him or her out of jail. These are codependent or enabling behaviors. This means that, without meaning to do so, family members are making it possible for the addict to continue to abuse alcohol or drugs.

RELATIONSHIPS

Codependency most often develops within families where someone suffers from a mental disorder, including addiction, depression, and anxiety disorders. Other family members, especially children, often come to believe that the enabling behaviors of codependency are part of a healthy relationship. According to Melody Beattie, author of *Codependent No More: How to Stop Controlling Others and Start Caring for Yourself,* people who have learned codependent behaviors are more likely to become involved in relationships with people who are unreliable, emotionally unavailable, or needy. The codependent person tries to control everything within the relationship without addressing his or her own needs or desires. This sets up the person for continued disappointment.

Even when those who are codependent encounter people with healthy boundaries, they still feel an overwhelming need to be needed. They are not likely to become seriously involved with anyone who sets realistic boundaries, because they believe a relationship requires that one partner be needy and the other enabling. Since people who are codependent connect the feeling of being needed with being loved, the absence of codependency may convince them that they are neither loved nor lovable. The result is a never-ending cycle unless they receive help. Without help, the same problems will plague each new relationship.

Q & A

Question: My brother wanted me to tell our mom he was in bed asleep, but he snuck out the window to go drinking with his friends. He does this a lot and I'm tired of lying. What should I do?

Answer: Lying for your brother doesn't help him, and it does hurt you. When you lie to your mother, you are damaging your relationship with her. When you sacrifice your relationship with your mother to lie for your brother, you are putting your brother's needs before your own. In addition, your brother is putting you in a unfair situation. It is your right to tell him you will not lie for him anymore. By being honest with him, you can also be honest with your mother—and you are taking care of yourself.

CODEPENDENCY AND ITS CONSEQUENCES

When friends or family members are suffering from a mental disorder like depression or anxiety, they may not be able to successfully care for themselves. Their neediness and vulnerability can spark enabling behaviors in the people around them. These behaviors may include calling in sick for a loved one, doing his or her work, or even assuming his or her responsibilities. These efforts are meant to help the person who is struggling with an illness. Yet the "helping" behaviors can delay the process of treatment. Those behaviors can also damage the person who is trying to help.

See also: Defense Mechanisms; Depression and Substance Abuse

FURTHER READING

Beattie, Melody. *Codependent No More: How to Stop Controlling Others and Start Caring for Yourself.* 2nd ed. Center City, Minnesota: Hazelden Information Education, January 1997.

———. *The New Codependency: Help and Guidance for Today's Generation.* New York: Simon & Schuster, 2009.

■ DEFENSE MECHANISMS

Psychological tools for avoiding or reducing anxiety. Defense mechanisms are commonly used to prevent emotional discomfort. If someone calls you worthless, it hurts. There are many ways of dealing with the insult: physically attacking the person, walking away to avoid hearing further insults, retaliating by insulting him or her, or trying to address what you believe may have prompted the person to insult you in the first place. These choices are all defense mechanisms—strategies that try to reduce the power of an incoming message of worthlessness. The aim is to make one feel more comfortable.

Defense mechanisms can help people through times of crisis. For example, individuals who are injured in a car crash or some other accident are sometimes unaware of what is happening around them.

Their body and mind seem to know there is a limit to how much they can handle at one time. Many people shift into a dreamlike state under these conditions. In this altered state they can absorb impressions, such as pain and fear, in a way that can help them survive.

COMMON DEFENSE MECHANISMS

Everyone uses defense mechanisms from time to time, but those who are suffering from depression or an anxiety disorder tend to use them to function in everyday life. Using these mechanisms excessively can make it difficult to see life as it really is. Under normal circumstances, people use defense mechanisms to cope with unpleasant aspects of reality, but relying on them too much can create serious problems. For example, they may make it harder to establish and maintain healthy relationships.

Denial '

Denial is a defense mechanism used to avoid dealing with a painful reality. Denial is said to be a **conscious** behavior because people are aware on some level that they are denying reality. A person may pretend or act as if problems don't exist, trying to protect themselves from an unpleasant situation such as addiction or abuse.

Q & A

Question: My friends tell me I'm in denial, but I think I don't have a problem. What should I do?

Answer: You are the only one who can know what is going on inside your head. However, if several people have noticed you are having trouble, it is a good idea to listen to what they have to say. Denial is a powerful defense mechanism. Some people liken denial to sitting in a room with an elephant and acting as if it were not there. If you think you might be using denial to cope with difficult situations in your life, contact an adult you trust, such as a teacher, a school counselor, a religious leader, or your doctor. You should ask him or her to help you find someone so you can talk to about your concerns.

Repression

Repression is a defense mechanism in which unacceptable or painful events, ideas, or wishes are pushed from awareness to the unconscious mind. Unlike denial, people who repress painful things are not aware they are using a defense mechanism.

Projection

Subconsciously attributing one's own thoughts, feelings or impulses onto somebody else, especially if the thought or feeling is unwanted, is called **projection**. It, too, is a defense mechanism. Suppose, for example, someone cheated on a test and blamed you for her wrongdoing. She may believe that you are responsible for her behavior. Projection can be so strong that people literally see problems in the behavior of others without realizing those problems actually exist within themselves. For example, some people who suffer from an addiction notice addictive behaviors in others but are unable to see their own addiction.

Fact Or Fiction?

If you believe you don't have a problem with drugs, you definitely don't have a problem.

The Facts: The problem with denial is that you don't easily see your own problem. You may need to experience quite a bit of difficulty before coming to terms with the truth. If you have a drug problem but are in denial about it, your grades may drop. You may start skipping classes because you are unprepared, oversleep every morning, or spend all of your time with buddies who are also getting high. These activities may lead to trouble with your teachers or your parents. It's possible that none of these problems is serious enough to shake your denial. If your life seems to be spiraling out of control and bad things keep happening, it might be a good idea to talk to someone about what's going on. Sometimes it is good to have someone else help you figure out if you might be in denial about something.

Reaction formation

An extreme and often dangerous defense mechanism is called **reaction formation**. Reaction formation occurs when someone adopts feelings, attitudes, or behaviors that are the opposite of desires and impulses he or she may unconsciously hold but find unacceptable. For example, if a person has feelings that are deeply upsetting, he or she may express exaggerated attitudes or behaviors that are the opposite of his or her real feelings. The exaggeration is an attempt to get rid of the unwanted feelings. For example, if someone is attracted to people of the same gender but believes homosexuality is morally wrong, he or she might loudly express disgust at anything related to homosexuality.

Rationalization

A **rationalization** is an attempt to justify or make tolerable feelings or behavior that otherwise would be offensive or objectionable. Rationalizations, both spoken and implied, are defense mechanisms that people use daily to maintain their self-esteem, the regard of others, and their private belief system. For example, if you are trying to lose weight and a friend wants to stop for ice cream, you may rationalize your sundae by telling yourself it's a special occasion. Rationalizations can also be used to deal with your own uncomfortable feelings or those of someone you care about. If you are having trouble falling asleep at night, you may attribute the problem to loud traffic or sounds inside your home rather than recognizing that an overwhelming worry is keeping you awake.

Displacement

A generally unhealthy way to rid oneself of emotions such as anger or hostility is through **displacement**. Displacement is the transfer of emotion from one subject or behavior to another that is less threatening. For example, a student who is angry at his or her teacher may not express any emotions at school but go home and yell at a younger sister or brother.

Compensation

Compensation is a defense mechanism that conceals undesirable shortcomings by exaggerating strengths. It stresses a personal strength to make up for a perceived deficiency. For example, some people who have trouble with schoolwork focus their time and energy on improving their athletic abilities rather than dealing with their grades.

FINDING BALANCE

Defense mechanisms are healthy in small doses. Overusing them, however, can result in a diminished ability to cope with life. People can become so dependent on them that they may lose sight of reality and suffer serious consequences as a result. They may no longer trust their own judgment, and those around them may also lose faith in them. Defense mechanisms are not the only way of coping with life.

Many people find it helpful to talk with a therapist to learn new and healthier coping techniques.

See also: Codependency; Depression and Substance Abuse

■ DEPRESSION, CAUSES OF

Chemical imbalances in the brain that cause a mental disorder, the most common symptoms or signs of which are long-lasting feelings of hopelessness and despair, poor concentration, lack of energy, and, sometimes, suicidal tendencies. No one knows for sure what causes the chemical imbalances that result in depression. That's why researchers and other scientists who study possible causes of depression refer to risk factors rather than causes. A risk factor refers to anything that may increase the probability that the illness will occur. Researchers try to identify and examine various risk factors in their search for direct causes of depression. An example of a risk factor for depression is cancer. Those who have cancer are more likely to suffer from depression than those who do not have the disease. So cancer can be called a risk factor for depression.

There are many risk factors for depression. A vulnerability to depression appears to run in some families, although not everyone at risk for depression gets depressed. Sometimes depression can be triggered by a traumatic event or life change. In other cases, depression may be the result of a medical illness, such as stroke or heart attack, or a side effect of medication taken for a medical condition not otherwise related to depression.

BIPOLAR DISORDER

Bipolar disorder is a mental disorder that includes feelings of extreme excitement or irritability termed "**mania**" in addition to the severe lows of depression. According to a 2002 report by the National Institute of Mental Health (NIMH), most scientists agree there is no single cause for bipolar disorder—rather, many factors act together to produce the illness.

Because bipolar disorder tends to run in families, researchers have been trying to determine if it is caused by specific genes—the stretches of DNA that contain hereditary information for a specific function. Genes influence how the body and mind work. There is no evidence that bipolar disorder, or other forms of depression, are entirely genetic. However, according to NIMH (2001), more than two-thirds of people with bipolar disorder have at least one close relative with the disorder or with depression. Studies of identical twins—twins who share the same genes—indicate that other factors also play a role in bipolar disorder (NIMH, 2002). If bipolar disorder were caused entirely by genes, the identical twin of someone with the illness would always develop it. Research has shown that this is not the case. However, a report by NIMH (1998) showed that if one twin has a bipolar disorder, the other twin is more likely than another sibling to develop the illness.

LEARNED BEHAVIORS

In studying how stressful events may lead to depression, researchers have developed a theory known as **learned helplessness.** According to this theory, those who experience chronic or repeated stressful events learn to feel helpless. This feeling of helplessness grows as they come to believe they have no control over the stressful situation.

People who are depressed often have negative beliefs about their ability to manage aspects of their lives, based on perceived failures in the past. Imagine an adolescent boy living with verbally abusive parents who call him stupid and claim he cannot do anything right. Over time the boy may come to believe his parents are right. As he begins to doubt his abilities and self-worth, he may begin to feel helpless and believe that most things are beyond his control. This feeling of helplessness may make him more vulnerable to depression at some point in his life.

Q & A

Question: More people seem to be depressed these days. Is the rate of depression increasing?

Answer: Depression has been recorded for centuries. "Melancholia," one of the earliest terms for depression, dates back to 460 B.C.E. and the Greek mathematician Hippocrates. According to the NIMH, some 60 million Americans are treated for depression. The Centers for Disease Control and Prevention (CDC) reports that of the 2.4 billion drugs prescribed in visits to doctors and hospitals in 2005, 118 million of these prescriptions were for antidepressants. Between 1995 and 2002, the most recent year for which statistics are available, the use of these drugs rose 48 percent, the CDC reported. However, it is unclear whether the rise is a result of an increase in depression or of an increased awareness of the disorder and easier access to treatment.

SPECIFIC EXPERIENCES

Specific events can trigger depression but usually only in people with psychological, inherited, or physical predispositions. A **predisposition** is a tendency of susceptibility to a disorder or illness. An example of a predisposition for depression would be a certain kind of brain chemistry. For those with a predisposition to depression, traumatic experiences, such as the death of a loved one, rape, or abuse, can lead to depression.

TEENS SPEAK

Remembering What Happened in My Childhood Was Difficult, But Worth It

When my therapist started asking me about the bus driver I had in elementary school, I felt numb. I pulled my knees into my chest on the couch and wrapped my arms around my legs. I wanted to get as small and tight as I could. I wanted to protect every part of me.

The words that came out of my mouth sounded normal and average, but they didn't match how I was feeling inside at all. I felt like someone else was doing the talking. Inside I felt like I couldn't move and that somehow I couldn't feel anything at all.

Luckily, my therapist noticed more than the words I was saying. We had been talking for several months about my life and my childhood. I was diagnosed with depression and was taking medication to treat it. My therapist said, "It seems like something is bothering you. Is it about the bus driver?"

I nodded. I couldn't answer her. She told me that was okay and that I only needed to say what I felt comfortable saying. After a while, I was able to talk and suddenly thoughts and memories about what happened when I was little started rushing back. I was lucky that I had a very safe place (my therapist's office) to talk about how I had been hurt.

I hadn't remembered any of it until then, but after talking about how I had been abused, my life started to get better. My therapist supported me and encouraged me to talk about all the feelings I had. I learned that the trauma of being hurt had affected how I dealt with everything else in my life. She said the experience could have contributed to why I was dealing with depression.

After I talked with my therapist about what had happened, I found it easier and easier to get along in life. Through therapy, medication, and healing my past, I am able to be happy again.

PSYCHOLOGICAL RISK FACTORS

Psychological risk factors play a significant role in the development of depression. A risk factor is a characteristic that makes it more likely a person will develop an illness.

Childhood experiences

People who become depressed have generally experienced more difficulties in childhood than those who do not become depressed. These difficulties may include sexual or physical abuse, a violent upbringing, separation from a parent, or mental illness in a parent. According to a report published by the National Association of Mental Illnesses (2004), a troubled childhood may trigger an early onset of depression.

DID YOU KNOW?

Young People and Depression

According to researchers at Harvard, depression among children increases at the rate of 23 percent each year.

Source: Harvard University, February 2002.

Stress

Stress is an emotionally disruptive or upsetting response to a challenging external influence. The relationship among stressful situations, a person's physical and emotional reactions to stress, and the onset of depression are complicated. Some people develop depression after a stressful event in their lives. Events such as the death of a loved one, the loss of a job, or the end of a relationship are often **traumatic** (extremely distressing, frightening, or shocking) and cause a great deal of stress. Stress can also occur as a result of positive events such as marriage, a move to a new city, or a new job. Both positive and negative events can contribute to the development of depression.

Other stressors—activities, experiences, or situations that cause stress—are loneliness or feelings of loss. The normal reaction to loss is grief. **Grief** is great sadness or sorrow and it usually ends on its own. It usually starts as a result of a specific event, such as the loss of a loved one, and eases over time. Because grief usually resolves itself, it generally does not require treatment. At times, the grieving process may not resolve itself and can develop into depression.

Stress may also be important in triggering future episodes of depression. Physical problems associated with stress include headaches, sleeplessness, and high blood pressure. As the body works to handle the stress, it may also become susceptible to various physical and mental ailments. So, if you spend a lot of time under serious levels of stress, you may be more at risk for developing depression even after the stressful events have passed.

Whether a stressful event itself can actually cause a person to become depressed is not known. At times everyone struggles with painful situations. More often than not, these changes do not result in depression. In fact, some people become depressed even when there is little or no stress in their lives. The same stressor may lead to depression in one person but not in another.

Pessimism

A **pessimist** is somebody who always expects the worst to happen in every situation. An **optimist** tends to feel hopeful and positive about life. A report in *Mayo Clinic Proceedings* (August 2002) noted that people who have optimistic outlooks generally live longer and healthier lives than pessimists.

Pessimists tend to blame themselves for whatever goes wrong and see events as negative, permanent, and unending. They have thoughts such as, "This is going to last forever, and it's going to ruin everything." In contrast, optimists often see harmful events as temporary and controllable. Pessimism may contribute to depression, or it may be a symptom of depression.

Fact Or Fiction?

People with depression are crazy.

The Facts: Depression is a mental disorder, also called a mental illness, involving a chemical imbalance in the brain. It is true that people suffering from depression may exhibit signs of instability and may behave differently than they did before the onset of the disorder. They may even perceive reality differently than people around them. However, they are not "crazy." The chemical imbalances that cause depression are just that, chemical imbalances. Depression is an illness, just as diabetes or cancer is, and the illness can be treated with professional help.

PHYSIOLOGICAL FACTORS

Many illnesses cause stress and make daily life difficult, which, in turn, can lead to depression. In some cases, a medical illness or drug treatment for an illness affects the brain directly, causing depression. Cancer is an example of a physiological condition that may indirectly lead to depression. Cancer may cause pain and interfere with the quality of life. These factors, in turn, can alter mood and views about life, causing depression.

Hormone-related diseases

The **hormonal system** which regulates the body's response to stress may be overactive in many people with depression. Also known as the endocrine system, the hormonal system consists of glands that secrete chemicals called **hormones** into the bloodstream. The system helps the body cope with stresses. Some studies suggest that the overactivation of the body's hormonal system might cause some people to become depressed. In fact, hormones and depression in women are closely related. Scientists have linked several hormones, including estrogen and cortisol, to depression in women.

Thyroid problems are commonly associated with depression. The **thyroid gland,** a butterfly-shaped gland which wraps around the front part of the throat, produces and releases hormones that help regulate body temperature, heart rate, and metabolism. If the gland releases too few hormones, in a condition referred to as an underactive thyroid, metabolism slows, which can cause depression.

Other conditions that stem from hormonal imbalances can also trigger depression. These include disorders of the parathyroid gland and of the adrenal glands, like **Cushing's disease** and **Addison's disease.** Both of these involve **cortisol.** Cortisol is a hormone that is released by the adrenal glands during periods of stress or agitation. Addison's disease occurs when the body does not produce enough cortisol, while Cushing's disease is a result of an oversupply of cortisol. Symptoms of both diseases include severe fatigue and muscle weakness, mimicking the symptoms of depression. Both diseases can also lead to depression.

Heart disease and stroke

Heart disease and depression go hand-in-hand. One study conducted by NIMH in Baltimore concluded that those who did not have heart disease but who had a history of depression were four times more likely to have a heart attack in the next 14 years than those who had no history of depression. In addition, researchers in Canada found that heart patients who were depressed were four times more likely to die within six months compared with those who were not depressed.

In addition, a Harvard Medical School study reported that about 50 percent of patients who survived a heart attack had some depressive symptoms, and up to 20 percent developed major depression. Moreover, people with post–heart attack depression were two to three times more likely to have another heart attack or die prematurely compared with heart attack victims who were not depressed.

The signs and symptoms of depression can be difficult to distinguish from the effects of **stroke,** which may include memory difficulties, irritability and fatigue. According to the National Institutes of Health (2002), depression affects up to 40 percent of stroke victims in the first two years following the stroke.

Cancer

According to the National Cancer Institute, depression affects about 25 percent of cancer patients. The diagnosis of depression can be difficult to make in people with cancer, due to the difficulty of separating the symptoms of depression from the side effects of medications or the symptoms of cancer.

Medical factors may also cause depression in cancer patients. Some medical causes of depression in cancer patients include uncontrolled pain, **anemia,** vitamin B_{12} or folate deficiency, fever, or abnormal levels of thyroid hormone or steroids in the blood. Medication usually relieves this type of depression more effectively than counseling, particularly if the medications that are causing the depression cannot be stopped without endangering the life of the patient.

Other diseases and conditions

Other medical conditions that may increase the risk of depression include vitamin deficiencies, **dementia** (including Alzheimer's disease, brain tumor, or brain injury), **obstructive sleep apnea,** Parkinson's disease, kidney disease, arthritis, HIV/AIDS infection, **chronic pain,** and **diabetes.**

Vitamins are organic substances that are essential to nutrition and normal metabolism. Those who don't receive enough of a particular vitamin in their body have a **vitamin deficiency.** Deficiencies of the vitamins thiamine (vitamin B_1), niacin, pyridoxine (B_6), or cobalamin (B_{12}) sometimes produce mental or emotional problems, including depression. For those who experience a depression caused by vitamin deficiencies, vitamin supplements are useful in treating the depression.

Dementia is a condition marked by a decline or loss of memory, reasoning power, and other intellectual faculties. Dementia may also affect a person's mood and personality. Dementia is caused by the destruction of brain cells. A head injury, a stroke, a brain tumor, or a disorder like Alzheimer's disease can damage brain cells. The Mayo Clinic (2001) reported that 40 percent of those with Alzheimer's disease will experience significant depression sometime during the course of their disease.

Q & A

Question: Is depression a normal part of growing old?

Answer: People once assumed that depression was a normal part of aging, but it is not. Most adults do not experience depression as they age. However, there are many illnesses that increase in frequency with age—heart disease and diabetes, for example. Although an elderly person should receive treatment for a physical problem or illness, a physical treatment may not address his or her emotional response to the illness. This is unfortunate, because those who experience depression may be allowed to suffer. Depression is—at any age—a treatable condition.

Obstructive sleep apnea is a disorder that causes restricted and often interrupted breathing patterns during sleep. According to the National Commission on Sleep Disorders Research, **sleep apnea** affects about 4 percent of men and about 2 percent of women. In addition, an estimated 40 million Americans suffer from **chronic** sleep disorders, while another 20 to 30 million experience sporadic sleep problems. Those numbers are expected to rise to 79 million for chronic suffers and 40 million for intermittent suffers by 2010, as the population ages. Disruptions in sleep caused by sleep apnea might result in problems in social settings and at work, which in turn might lead to depression.

Chronic pain is pain that persists or reoccurs for indefinite periods. According to Harvard researchers, people who experience chronic pain are three times more likely to have psychiatric problems, including mood or anxiety disorders and depression. In addition, people who are already depressed are three times more likely to develop chronic pain problems. Researchers found that a person with a history of major depression was three times more likely than average to have a first migraine attack. A person with a history of migraine headaches was five times more likely than average to have a first bout of depression. Depression in a patient with chronic pain might be left untreated because of a sense that it is somehow appropriate that the pain sufferer be depressed.

Diabetes is a chronic condition caused by the body's inability to process sugar, usually due to a lack of insulin. Most of the food you eat is broken down into **glucose.** Glucose is a form of sugar that is the main source of fuel for the body. After digestion, glucose passes into the bloodstream. **Insulin,** a hormone produced by the pancreas, converts glucose to energy. Without insulin, glucose builds up in the blood, and the body loses its main source of fuel.

In 2008, the *Journal of the American Medical Association* reported that people with diabetes are more likely to be depressed. About 21 million people suffer from diabetes, while 30 million have symptoms of depression. According to the study, those patients who had symptoms of depression are 30 percent more likely to develop diabetes than people who are not depressed.

The NIMH reports that the chances of becoming depressed increase as complications from diabetes worsen. Depression leads to poorer physical and mental functioning, so a person with diabetes who develops depression is less likely to follow a required diet or medication plan.

The exact relationship between depression and diabetes is unclear. Depression may develop because of stress, but the NIMH reports that depression also may result from the metabolic effects of diabetes on the brain. According to the NIMH, studies suggest that people with diabetes who have a history of depression are more likely to develop complications from diabetes than those without such a history.

DRUG USE

The relationship between depression and substance abuse is complicated. Dependence on alcohol or drugs can increase the risk of depression. According to researchers at University of California–Davis, it is estimated that 25 percent of people with alcohol or drug abuse problems also have depression.

In addition to substance abuse, the use of some commonly prescribed or over-the-counter medications can cause depression. The following types of medications are known to cause depression:

- drugs for high blood pressure
- drugs for heart disease
- painkillers
- drugs for stomach and intestinal problems
- anticonvulsants
- sedatives and sleeping pills
- drugs for Parkinson's disease
- cancer chemotherapy drugs
- oral contraceptives
- antibiotics

Proper diagnosis of depression should include a discussion of all drug use.

GENETICS AND FAMILY HISTORY

In some families, depression occurs in generation after generation. This suggests that some forms of depression, including bipolar disorder, may be inherited. However, depression also occurs in people who have no family history of the disorder. So, while it has been known for a long time that depression can "run in families," it is not known if the cause is genetic or environmental. Certain genes may be responsible for causing depression. Or, particularly stressful factors in some families may increase the risk of depression. An example would be an abusive household.

See also: Depression and Families; Depression, Symptoms of; Genetics of Mood and Anxiety Disorders; Risk Factors for Depression

FURTHER READING
Swartz, Karen L. *Depression and Anxiety.* Johns Hopkins White Papers. New York: Rebus, Inc., 2004.
Zucker, Faye, and Joan E. Huebl. *Beating Depression: Teens Find Light at the End of the Tunnel.* Scholastic Choices. New York: Children's Press, 2007.

■ DEPRESSION, SYMPTOMS OF

The most common symptoms of depression are long-lasting feelings of hopelessness and despair. Anyone who experiences sadness might say he or she feels "depressed." But feeling sad is different from the mental disorder called depression. Feeling blue or sad, especially while undergoing a difficult life experience, is normal. When sad feelings continue a long time, appear for no reason, or begin to affect many aspects of life—eating, sleeping, school, relationships—they may be symptoms, or signs, of depression.

Symptoms of depression may be physical, mental, and emotional. They include

- ■ feeling sad or depressed
- ■ losing interest in pleasurable activities such as sports or hanging out with friends
- ■ losing or gaining weight without trying
- ■ sleeping too much or too little
- ■ feeling tired, weak, or slowed down most of the time
- ■ feeling hopeless, guilty, or worthless
- ■ thinking about death and dying or suicide

The National Mental Health Association (NMHA) has a Web site with a confidential depression screening exam available to anyone who would like to take the test at http://depression-screening.org. The short test can help people decide whether their symptoms are related to depression.

Q & A

Question: If I am depressed, where can I go for help?

Answer: If you are concerned about depression, you should talk to someone who can help—a psychologist, your school counselor, teacher, school nurse, your parents or other trusted family member, your family doctor, a religious advisor, or a professional at a mental health center.

PHYSICAL SYMPTOMS

Although depression is a mental disorder, it has physical symptoms. Because symptoms of depression are often physical, diagnosing the disorder can be challenging. The sufferer may mistake the physical symptoms of depression for those associated with another problem. Physical symptoms of depression include

- changes in eating habits. Those with depression may not feel hungry and may lose weight without trying. Or they may overeat and gain weight.
- changes in sleeping patterns. Those who experience depression may have trouble falling asleep at night, wake up frequently during the night, or wake up early in the morning and not be able to get back to sleep. Or they may sleep too much and spend much of the day in bed.
- exhaustion without an obvious cause. People who are depressed may have a low energy level and feel tired all the time. Their body movements may slow down, and they may talk more slowly.

Other physical symptoms that are commonly associated with depression include headaches, digestive disorders, or chronic pain (pain that continues over months or years).

Fact Or Fiction?

It is unusual for teenagers to experience depression.

The Facts: Being depressed for a few days is common. In fact, 90 percent of teenagers experience a day or two of depression. If the depression lasts for more than a few weeks, however, they should talk with someone about it.

MENTAL AND EMOTIONAL SYMPTOMS

The mental and emotional symptoms of depression are the best-known symptoms. However, as with the physical symptoms, it is not always easy to recognize depression based on mental and emotional symptoms alone. For example, someone who is easily irritated may blame his or her irritation on annoying situations rather than seeing the irritation as a symptom of depression. Mental and emotional symptoms of depression include

- **long-lasting sadness.** Those with depression are likely to feel blue, sad, or empty. They may cry all of the time or feel numb—neither happy nor sad.

- **irritability.** They may be easily irritated and get upset over things that never used to bother them.

- **feelings of anxiety.** They may be unusually nervous, worried, or preoccupied with minor concerns—always making a big deal out of little things. They may feel restless or experience stomach upset.

- **loss of interest or pleasure in life.** People with depression may lose the ability to find pleasure in people, hobbies, or activities they previously enjoyed.

- **neglect of responsibilities.** Those who normally did well at work or school activities may find themselves falling behind at their job or cutting classes.

- **neglect of personal care.** People with depression often lack the energy to bathe regularly or maintain their usual routines of personal hygiene.

PERSONALITY CHANGES

Many people complain that they lose their old personalities while suffering from depression. Those who are depressed often have little enthusiasm and usually are not interested in being with other people. When the depression is resolved, the individual's old personality should gradually return.

CLINICAL SYMPTOMS

A symptom is clinical if it can be observed. Psychiatrists and other mental health professionals don't have to rely solely on what a patient tells them to make a diagnosis. They also look for symptoms of depression that can be observed objectively no matter what the patient says. Such symptoms include changes in personal hygiene, level of irritability, or speech patterns.

BIPOLAR DISORDER

Bipolar disorder causes dramatic mood swings—from overly "high" or irritable to sad and hopeless, and back again. Often, people with bipolar disorders experience relatively calm periods between the highs and the lows. Extreme changes in energy and behavior accompany these changes in mood. The highs are referred to as episodes of **mania** and the lows as periods of depression. The depression associated with bipolar disorders has symptoms similar to those of other forms of depression.

Mania is an abnormally and persistently elevated (high) mood or irritability accompanied by at least three of the following symptoms:

- overly inflated self-esteem
- decreased need for sleep
- increased talkativeness
- racing thoughts
- distractibility
- increased goal-directed activity such as shopping
- physical agitation
- excessive involvement in risky behaviors or activities

SEASONAL AFFECTIVE DISORDER (SAD)

Some people suffer from symptoms of depression during the winter months. This may be a sign of seasonal affective disorder (SAD). SAD is a mental disorder associated with depression and related to seasonal variations of light.

According to the Substance Abuse and Mental Health Services Administration (SAMHSA), SAD was first noted before 1845, but was not officially named until the early 1980s. As seasons change, the body's "biological clock" or **circadian rhythm** shift, due partly to changes in sunlight patterns. These shifts can cause the body's biological clock to be "out of sync" with normal daily routines. SAMHSA reports that the most difficult months for SAD sufferers are January and February, and young people and women are at highest risk.

DYSTHYMIC DISORDER

A person who suffers from a variety of depressive symptoms for at least two years is generally diagnosed as having a dysthymic disorder. Dysthymic disorders are often difficult to diagnose because the symptoms are hard to distinguish from major depressive disorder. Those who suffer from dysthymic disorder experience changes in the way they sleep and eat, often have low energy, and are routinely fatigued. They also may experience low self-esteem and poor concentration. Because they might feel pessimistic or inadequate, they might want to withdraw socially.

The disorder usually occurs during the teenage years or early adulthood. Because its arrival is so early in a person's development, and causes feelings of inadequacy that can interfere with the person's social life, it can change an individual's personality. Because such individuals never experienced a normal life as teens or young adults, those suffering from the affliction might just resign themselves to feeling pessimistic about life. As a result, they might not seek treatment until the depression becomes even more severe. According to the University of Michigan, 10 percent of those suffering from dysthymic disorder develop major symptoms of depression. Some have said that they have been depressed for decades before seeking treatment.

DIAGNOSTIC PROCEDURES

Diagnostic procedures are the methods used to identify a condition or illness. The first step in diagnosing depression is often a physical exam by a medical doctor.

Certain prescription medications and some medical conditions such as a viral infection may cause symptoms identical to those associated with depression. The doctor will try to rule out these possibilities through a checkup and, possibly, laboratory tests. If a physical cause for the depression is ruled out, he or she may call for a psychological evaluation.

Health-care professionals are very careful when evaluating clients for depression. It takes more than a feeling of sadness to justify a diagnosis of depression. Therefore they take the time to gather as much information as possible before deciding that a patient is experiencing depression. In addition to a medical evaluation and an interview, they look for and evaluate specific symptoms of depression.

Mental health professionals have grouped the symptoms of disorders such as depression into a reference work called the *Diagnostic and Statistical Manual of Mental Disorders, Fourth Edition (DSM-IV)* (2001). Professionals use it to aid in diagnosing various mental disorders, including depression.

A good diagnostic evaluation includes questions about symptoms, such as when they started, how long they have lasted, how severe they are, whether they have occurred previously, and if so, whether the symptoms were treated and what treatment was given. The doctor usually asks about the individual's use of alcohol and drugs (and the frequency of that use) as well as about thoughts of death or suicide. There are also likely to be questions about whether other family members have suffered from depression. If these family members were treated, the doctor will want to know what treatments they received and which were most effective.

ASSISTANCE WITH THE SYMPTOMS

Depression has a wide range of symptoms, both emotional and physical. The symptoms of depression are easy to confuse with other disorders if they are taken separately. When symptoms become severe enough that the tasks of daily life are difficult, the assistance of a professional diagnostician is essential.

See also: Mental Health Professionals, Types of; Risk Factors for Depression

FURTHER READING

Hamil, Sara. *My Feeling Better Workbook: Help for Kids Who Are Sad and Depressed.* Oakland, Calif.: New Harbinger Publications, 2008.

■ DEPRESSION AND ADDICTION

See: Defense Mechanisms; Depression and Alcoholism; Depression and Substance Abuse

■ DEPRESSION AND ALCOHOLISM

Depression, a mental disorder caused by a chemical imbalance in the brain, the most common symptoms of which are long-lasting feelings of hopelessness and despair; and alcoholism, an illness marked by consumption of alcoholic beverages at levels that interfere with daily living. Many people who suffer from depression also suffer from alcoholism.

Sometimes people who experience depression may try to "self-medicate" by drinking heavily in an effort to feel better. Such behavior is risky for several reasons. Alcohol is a **depressant.** Therefore it can intensify depression. Depression combined with alcohol is not only dangerous—it can be deadly.

According to a 2004 report of the National Alliance for the Mentally Ill (NAMI), the combination of mental disorders and substance abuse, such as alcoholism, is so common that medical professionals now expect to find it. Studies show that more than half of young people who abuse alcohol and other substances also have a diagnosable mental disorder. The link between depression and alcoholism is well established, but the reasons for the connection are not well understood.

COMORBIDITY

Comorbidity is the presence of a second disease or condition that influences the care or treatment of another condition. The term is used interchangeably with such terms as dual diagnosis, co-occurring illnesses, concurrent disorders, comorbid disorders, co-occurring disorders, or dual disorders.

According to a 2004 report by the National Mental Health Association:

- ■ Thirty-seven percent of alcohol abusers also have at least one other serious mental disorder.
- ■ Of all people diagnosed with mental disorders, 29 percent abuse either alcohol or drugs.

Comorbid illnesses may occur at the same time or one after the other. The fact that two illnesses are comorbid, however, does not necessarily imply that one is the cause of the other, even if one occurs first.

SYMPTOMS AND RECOVERY

At times the symptoms of alcoholism and depression can overlap and even mask each other, making diagnosis and treatment more difficult. Symptoms of alcoholism that overlap with symptoms of depression include:

- drinking alcohol excessively
- feeling overly tired, exhausted
- sleep difficulties (too much or not enough)
- gastrointestinal discomfort (nausea, diarrhea, ulcers)
- headaches
- feeling emotionally "numb"
- eating difficulties (too much or not enough)

Physical effects of alcohol

Alcohol slows down the **central nervous system,** the parts of the brain and spinal cord that control and coordinate most bodily functions. Common short-term effects of alcohol use include decreased inhibitions, relaxation, talkativeness, and sociability. Further effects include blurred vision, impaired hearing, and loss of coordination. Higher doses of alcohol often cause a loss of muscle control, which leads to slurred speech, further loss of vision, and wobbly legs. Abusing alcohol may lead to loss of consciousness or death.

Alcohol abuse can also have long-term effects. These include cancer of the mouth and throat, stomach ulcers (raw sores in the stomach walls), **gastritis** (an inflammation of the stomach walls), and diarrhea.

The liver can handle only so much alcohol at one time. An overloaded liver can suffer in a number of ways. Fatty liver, alcoholic hepatitis, and **cirrhosis** are examples of liver diseases caused by excessive alcohol use. Cirrhosis occurs when so much of the liver is scarred that it can't process and clean the blood as it normally would.

Other common physical effects include **anemia,** skin problems, and diminished physical fitness. Anemia is a condition in which the body produces too few red blood cells. Since red blood cells deliver oxygen to the organs and muscles, anemia results in fatigue. It generally requires medical attention. Many or most of these physical effects are similar to the physical effects of depression.

Treatment

Because of the overlapping symptoms, a person may sincerely try to recover from one illness while not acknowledging the other. Without specific treatment, a co-occurring mental disorder may recur. The recurrence may, in turn, lead to further alcohol abuse. Over time, the lack of progress toward recovery on both fronts may trigger feelings of failure and alienation.

When both depression and alcoholism are diagnosed, both should be treated simultaneously. Usually, treatment for comorbid depression and alcoholism is very much like treatment for dependence on alcohol alone. The first step in treatment is detoxification—the process of safely getting alcohol out of the body. Ideally, detoxification should take place under medical supervision. It can take a few days to a week or more, depending on the length of time the alcohol abuse has occurred.

Until recently, detoxification meant a painful and sometimes life-threatening "cold turkey" withdrawal. Doctors now are able to give hospitalized alcoholics carefully chosen medications to ease withdrawal symptoms. Thus, when detoxification is done under medical supervision, it is safer and less traumatic.

Treatment for alcoholism and depression often involves individual or group therapy, education about alcoholism and depression, exercise, proper nutrition, and participation in a 12-step recovery program such as Alcoholics Anonymous. The idea is not just to stop using alcohol, but to learn to enjoy life without it.

In therapy, alcoholics and people with depression learn healthier behaviors and social interactions. The goal is to avoid actions that may cause a relapse and to recognize the symptoms of depression if they recur.

Treatment for depression also often includes the use of medicines called antidepressants. Fluoxetine (Prozac), a kind of antidepressant called a **selective serotonin reuptake inhibitor** (SSRI), has actually been effective in decreasing depressive symptoms and the level of alcohol consumption in depressed alcoholics.

SUICIDE

According to researchers at Johns Hopkins Bloomberg School of Public Health, the suicide rate in the United States is on the rise.

Researchers found that from 1999 to 2005, the overall suicide rate in the United States rose 0.7 percent. The suicide rate for middle-aged white women increased 3.9 percent, while the suicide rate for middle-aged white men was 2.7 percent. During that same period, the suicide rate declined for African Americans and remained stable for Asians and Native Americans.

The report was published on October 21, 2008, in the *American Journal of Preventive Medicine*. According to the report, the majority of those who commit suicide prefer to use a firearm. However, 22 percent of all suicides occurred as a hanging or suffocation.

It was also found that men were more likely to hang or suffocate themselves than women. Researchers said that in 2004, suicide was the 11th leading cause of death in the United States, accounting for 32,439 fatalities. According to the National Institute of Mental Health, eight to 25 people attempt suicide each year for every suicide death. Alcohol abuse makes the problem worse. Alcohol increases the risk of suicide by deepening depression and affecting the ability of people to make decisions. Even non–problem drinkers had an elevated suicide rate. A Harvard study says the odds of a drinker committing suicide are two times greater than for a person who does not drink. According to the National Center for Health Statistics, alcoholism is a factor in 30 of all successful suicides.

FAMILY AND FRIENDS

In the rehabilitation for alcoholism and treatment for depression, the greater a family's understanding of the problems, the better the chances the patient will have a lasting recovery.

It is essential that friends and family stop enabling. Those who enable act in ways that help or encourage a loved one's drinking. For instance, a woman whose husband routinely drinks too much might call in sick for him when he is too drunk to go to work. When family and friends participate in the recovery program, they learn how to stop enabling. If they act on what they've learned, the recovering alcoholic is much less likely to relapse.

Regarding the treatment for depression, friends and family should be calm and understanding, rather than frightened or critical. They should be warm and open, instead of cool or cautious. It is fine to ask the person matter-of-factly about his or her treatment, though it is important to talk about more than just the disorder.

If someone you care about seems to be suffering from alcoholism or depression, encourage him or her to acknowledge the problem and seek professional help. Suggest a professional evaluation with a licensed physician, preferably at a medical center that's equipped to treat alcoholism and mental disorders. A little encouragement may be all it takes.

See also: Codependency; Depression and Substance Abuse; Suicide

FURTHER READING
Schab, Lisa, M. *Beyond the Blues: A Workbook to Help Teens Overcome Depression.* Oakland, Calif.: New Harbinger Publications, 2008.

■ DEPRESSION AND FAMILIES
Depression—a mental disorder caused by a chemical imbalance in the brain, the most common symptoms or signs of which are long-lasting feelings of hopelessness and despair, poor concentration, lack of energy, and, sometimes, suicidal tendencies—and its impact on families. Depression changes people. Those changes in a family member can be confusing for others in the family who don't understand what is happening to their loved one. For that reason, the changes that take place in a person who is experiencing depression can have a serious impact on an entire family.

DEPRESSION AFFECTS FAMILIES
Some people who are depressed show subtle signs and symptoms months or years before they are diagnosed and treated. This early phase before treatment can be difficult for everyone in the family. Some people who experience depression withdraw and isolate themselves. They may start to abuse alcohol or drugs. Still others may become irritable and moody and have angry outbursts. Being around someone who is constantly withdrawn, moody, or angry can be upsetting.

Episodes of depression can be triggered by stressful events like unemployment, financial worries, illness, or marital problems. In these cases, the family has to deal with these very real problems in addition to dealing with a loved one who is depressed.

When family members are confused as to why the behavior of a relative has suddenly changed, they may become angry. Their anger may intensify family problems.

TEENS SPEAK

Living with Family Members Suffering from Depression

My mom and I are best friends, but a while ago she started acting differently. Instead of wanting to do things with me, she always wanted to be alone. I couldn't believe how much she slept. When I came home from school, she was asleep. When it was time for dinner, she was asleep. I didn't know anyone could sleep so much.

I have always loved my mom, even when she just stayed in her room. But I missed the fun times we used to have. I could still talk to her about stuff, but sometimes she seemed more like a robot than a person. I missed the connection we used to have. I wanted my mom back.

I could tell something was really wrong when she stopped eating. She started looking much thinner, like she hadn't eaten in a long time. She didn't look healthy.

My father convinced her to get some professional help. She finally decided that, for my sake, she would talk to a professional. She started seeing a therapist every week and started taking medication. The pills were to help the chemicals in her brain balance out.

After a while, Mom was a lot better. I felt like she was a human again, not a robot. She was a lot livelier and I liked her again.

She started cooking and doing activities with me. We started talking again and having fun like we used to. She had more friends over. We were finally close again like we used to be.

It was hard when she was so sick, but I'm glad she started to take care of herself. I know she might have to see a therapist and take medication for a long time, but it's so good to have my mom back!

GENETICS AND FAMILY HISTORY

A **genetic** disorder is an illness that is inherited or runs in families. Genes are passed from parent to child. Shared genes give family members similar traits, such as hair color and eye color. Close relatives of people with depression are more likely to develop the mental disorder than people without such a family history. Keep in mind, however, that other factors—including difficult family relationships, serious illness, major loss or change, or substance abuse—can also cause or complicate depression.

Those who have close relatives with depression may have inherited a tendency to develop the illness. For example, if one identical twin has depression, the other twin has a 70 percent chance of developing the disorder, according to a 1999 report by the American Psychiatric Association. Because of the increased risk, learning if there is a history of depression in your family may be useful. However, having family members with depression does not necessarily mean that you will become depressed.

CHILDREN

Even very young children can suffer from depression. According to researchers at Harvard Medical Center, childhood depression is rapidly increasing by 23 percent each year. According to some studies, 10 percent of children suffer from depression that is so severe it affects their daily lives.

Depression in children is usually more difficult to diagnose than it is in adults. Because normal behaviors vary from one childhood stage to another, determining whether a child is just going through a "phase" or is suffering from depression can be difficult. Irritability, anxiety, and complaints of boredom are normal parts of childhood but can also be indicators of depression.

The following list suggests how children of various ages might exhibit depression.

A preschooler with depression may

- be listless;
- be uninterested in playing; or
- cry easily and frequently.

A child in elementary school with depression may

- be listless and moody;
- be more irritable than he or she has been in the past;
- be easily discouraged;
- complain of being bored;
- be distant with family and friends;
- have difficulty with schoolwork; or
- talk about death often.

If you know a child who might be depressed, there are resources listed in the Hotlines and Help Sites section.

Q & A

Question: Is it true that if I have depression, I won't succeed in school, at work, or in relationships?

Answer: Having depression does not mean you will not succeed. In fact, many well-known and highly respected figures are among the millions of people who experience depression. Abraham Lincoln, Winston Churchill, and Vincent Van Gogh are three of the many historic figures known to have suffered from serious depression.

Fact Or Fiction?

It's normal for teenagers to be moody; teens don't suffer from "real" depression.

The Facts: Depression is more than just being moody—it is a physiological illness that can affect people of any age, including teens. Approximately 5 percent of teens become seriously depressed each year.

PREVENTIVE ACTIONS FOR TEENS

Losing hope, feeling alone, or believing that something is permanently wrong with you, your family, or your life is a heavy weight to bear. Preventing severe or even mild depression begins with understanding the problem. A school counselor can be a helpful resource for information on teen depression.

Seeking professional help is important because depression rarely goes away on its own and it can have fatal consequences. Untreated depression can lead to suicide. The NIMH estimated in the year 2000 that about 60 percent of people who committed suicide had a mental disorder such as depression. Some 80–90 percent of mental disorders are treatable using medication and other therapies, according to a 1999 report from the Surgeon General.

Discussions with people you trust are important. Talk to a good friend, a family member (your parent or guardian, if possible), a religious advisor, a friend's parent, a coach, or a school counselor. Look for people you can trust and let them into your life. Finding a safe way to discuss your feelings can help you make sense of them and hopefully find solutions to your problems.

Staying physically healthy is also a way to help prevent depression. Regular exercise, a balanced diet, and good-quality sleep can help decrease the chances of developing depression or anxiety disorders.

PREVALENCE AMONG TEENS

Although mental disorders like depression often begin in childhood, there is a sharp increase in the number of people affected at adolescence. According to the federal Center for Mental Health Services, population studies show that at any point in time, 10 to 15 percent of children and adolescents have *some* symptoms of depression. A report by the National Mental Health Association (2004) notes that once a young person has experienced a bout of depression, he or she is at risk of developing it again within the next five years.

ECONOMICS

Studies suggest that there may be a connection between socioeconomic class and depression. An article in *Health Care Financing Review* (2001) supports those findings. It stated that being of limited means is a major risk factor for depression. According to a report in *Well-Connected* (2003), actual poverty or unemployment increases the duration of an existing depression but doesn't seem to cause it. Feelings of financial insecurity both cause and prolong depression.

The Agency for Healthcare Research and Quality (2001) reported that women who are poor, have little formal schooling, and are on welfare or are unemployed are more likely to experience depression than women in the general population.

DEPRESSION IN THE FAMILY

When a family member suffers from depression, the whole family is affected. Some family members actively try to help their loved one. Others may find other coping mechanisms to deal with the painful experience of living with someone who is depressed. Although there is no data showing a direct genetic cause of depression, people who have a family history of depression are more likely to become depressed. Anyone in a family can suffer from depression, but it is hardest to diagnose the disorder in young children. If you suspect a loved one is suffering from depression, encourage him or her to get professional help, because depression is a treatable disorder.

See also: Codependency; Depression, Causes of

FURTHER READING

Kantory, Martin, M.D. *Lifting the Weight: Understanding Depression in Men, Its Causes and Solutions.* Westport, Conn.: Praeger Publishers, 2007.

■ DEPRESSION AND SUBSTANCE ABUSE

A mental disorder caused by a chemical imbalance in the brain, the most common symptoms or signs of which are long-lasting feelings of hopelessness and despair, poor concentration, lack of energy, and which is sometimes accompanied by the excessive use of substances such as alcohol or drugs. People who suffer from depression are more likely to abuse substances such as alcohol and drugs than those who do not have a mental disorder.

Depression can increase the risk of abusing substances. In fact, the National Mental Health Association (2004) reported that one in three people with depression also suffer from some form of substance abuse or dependence. Those who experience depression may try to "self-medicate" by taking drugs or drinking heavily in an effort to feel better. Such behavior is risky for several reasons. Alcohol and a number of other drugs are **depressants**—they quiet or depress the nervous system. They can therefore intensify depression. Also, many of the illegal drugs available today are more dangerous, numerous, potent, and affordable than they were a few decades ago. As a result, the use of these substances may quickly lead to **addiction**—psychological, emotional, or physical dependence on the effects of a drug—and further health problems.

RATES

Depression contributes to the serious problems associated with substance abuse. However, the relationship between the two disorders is complicated. Rather than one disorder causing the other, depression and substance abuse often occur simultaneously. Doctors often refer to this phenomenon as **comorbid** conditions. According to *Mental Health: A Report of the Surgeon General* (1999), approximately 15 percent of all adults who have any kind of mental illness in any given year also experience a substance abuse disorder. A similar report in *Well'-Connected* estimated that 25 percent of people with alcohol or drug abuse problems also have depression.

The U.S. Surgeon General reports that approximately 15 percent of all adults who have any kind of mental illness in any given year will also experience a substance abuse disorder. People with depression are as likely to abuse substances as substance abusers are likely to become depressed. However, a report in the *Clinical Psychological Review*

DID YOU KNOW?

Depression and Addiction

Depression can lead to substance abuse, and abuse can lead to addiction. In 2005, about 10.8 million people in the United States between the ages of 12 and 20 (28.2 percent) reported drinking alcohol in the past month. In addition, nearly 7.2 million people (18.8 percent) were binge drinkers, and 2.3 million (6.0 percent) drank heavily.

Source: U.S. Department of Health and Human Services Office of Applied Studies, 2005.

(Swendsen, Merikangas 2000) observed that teenagers are more likely to abuse substances first and then develop depression than the reverse.

TYPES OF SUBSTANCES

There are four major groups of drugs: stimulants, depressants, narcotics, and psychedelics.

Stimulants reduce appetite, provide the feeling of a "lift" or "high," and give an exaggerated sense of increased energy. Examples of stimulants include amphetamines (speed), cocaine, caffeine, and nicotine.

Depressants quiet and slow the nervous system. They are often used to reverse the effects of stimulant abuse. These drugs include alcohol, tranquilizers, and inhalants (sniffers or huffers).

Narcotics, when used legitimately, bring relief from pain and induce sleep. They also cause a short-term sense of well-being. Excessive doses may lead to unconsciousness, coma, and death. Examples of narcotics are heroin, opium, morphine, and codeine.

Psychedelics change one's perception of reality. Time seems to slow down or speed up. Hallucinations and strange thought processes may occur. Included in this group of drugs are LSD, PCP, marijuana, and ecstasy. Like narcotics, psychedelics offer the dangerous illusion that they provide an escape from reality.

While substance abuse often consists of illegal drug use, legal drugs may be abused as well. Certain prescription drugs—particularly narcotics, depressants, and stimulants—can, when abused, alter the brain's activity and lead to dependence and addiction. According to the National Institute of Health, 20 percent of those living in the United States use prescription drugs for nonmedical purposes. According to a 2007 survey conducted for the National Institute on Drug Abuse, 15 percent of high school seniors abuse prescription drugs, especially painkillers such as OxyContin and Vicodin.

According to the National Institute on Drug Abuse, prescription drug abuse has increased as the drugs become easier to obtain. In the United States, the prescriptions written for stimulants increased from 5 million in 1991 to almost 35 million in 2007. In addition, the number of prescriptions for opioid painkillers, such as Oxycontin and Vicodin, increased from 40 million in 1991 to 180 million in 2007.

How do some people get hold of other peoples' prescription drugs? Most doctors write prescriptions for people who truly need the medicine. Many households, however, contain drawers and cabinets filled with leftover drugs. Some individuals, especially teens, will raid the drawers and cabinets looking for a cheap high. Because prescription drugs have medical uses, children often believe wrongly that these drugs are a safe alternative to street drugs.

Pain relievers are also popular among drug addicts. According to a U.S. Department of Health and Human Services survey, in 2004, 4.4 million Americans 12 years old or older reported abusing pain relievers in the month before being questioned. Almost 5 percent, or 11.3 million people, had abused pain relievers in the year prior to the survey. When asked, 31.8 million people, or 13.2 percent, said they had abused prescription drugs in their lifetime. Those using pain relievers for nonmedical reasons jumped from 29.6 million in 2002 to 31.8 million in 2004. OxyContin seems to be the drug of choice for many who do not medically need the drug. The use of OxyContin increased from 1.9 million people in 2002 to 3.1 million people in 2004.

EFFECTS OF SUBSTANCE ABUSE

In general, the effects associated with substance abuse are both physical and mental. They can be short- or long-term. Short-term effects include disorientation, impaired judgment, and a loss of touch with reality. Long-term effects can include brain damage or death.

The damaging effects of substance abuse are caused both directly, by the drug itself, and indirectly, by the way the drug is taken. When drugs are injected into the bloodstream, diseases such as HIV/AIDS and hepatitis can occur through the use of dirty syringes. If the drugs are taken through the nasal passages, damage can occur to the nose and sinus cavities. Drugs taken orally can irritate and damage the **gastrointestinal** tract, and inhaling drugs can lead to an increase in the rates of lung disease.

Physical effects of alcohol

Alcohol is a depressant—it slows down the action of the **central nervous system.** The central nervous system consists of the parts of the brain and spinal cord that control and coordinate most functions of the body and mind. Common short-term effects of alcohol include decreased inhibitions, relaxation, talkativeness, and sociability. Other effects are distorted vision and hearing and impaired coordination. Higher doses of alcohol can lead to a loss of control that is evidenced by slurred speech, blurred vision, and wobbly legs. Abusing alcohol may also lead to loss of consciousness or death.

Physical effects of other drugs

The negative effects of long-term marijuana use include a loss of **short-term memory**. Short-term memory is often called working memory. It includes information temporarily stored as it is being processed. For example, suppose you go to the store to buy a loaf of bread. When you arrive at the store, you can't remember what you came to purchase— a lapse in short-term memory. The National Institute on Drug Abuse (NIDA) reported in 1998 that using marijuana could cause problems with not only short-term memory but also learning, thinking, and problem-solving.

Used over a long period of time, marijuana can affect personality, leading to an emotional flatness and loss of interest in the world. According to the NIDA (2003), marijuana use can make it more difficult to handle the everyday frustrations of life. The NIDA (2003) reported that depression, anxiety, and personality disturbances are all associated with marijuana use; marijuana use has the potential to cause problems in daily life or make existing problems worse. Because marijuana compromises the ability to learn and remember information, the more a person uses marijuana the more likely he or she is likely to fall behind in acquiring intellectual, job, or social skills.

Cocaine, an addictive stimulant drug derived from the leaves of the coca plant, constricts the blood vessels. When cocaine is converted into hard or flaky white rocks intended for smoking, it is called **crack cocaine**. The physical effects of cocaine and crack are similar: The blood pressure rises, the pupils dilate, and the heartbeat increases by up to 50 percent. Using cocaine and crack can result in severe weight loss, **insomnia** (inability to sleep), and **psychosis** (a disorder that includes hallucinations and delusions). Snorting cocaine powder can irritate the nose's mucus membranes and even cause ulcers in the nose.

Speed is an amphetamine drug also known as an "upper." In its various forms—including diet pills—speed has a quick and violent effect on the body. It can result in a faster heartbeat, a rise in blood pressure, and often feelings of anxiety or nervousness. Using these stimulants can lead to unhealthy weight loss. These drugs can also contribute to heart failure, loss of coordination, and psychosis.

Depressants like barbiturates, sedatives, and tranquilizers (including alcohol) can cause drowsiness, confusion, mood swings, poor coordination, and, in some people, extreme agitation.

See also: Codependency; Related Disorders

FURTHER READING
Schab, Lisa M. *Beyond the Blues: A Workbook to Help Teens Overcome Depression.* Oakland, Calif.: New Harbinger Publications, 2008.
Westermeyer, Joseph J., et al., eds. *Integrated Treatment for Mood and Substance Use Disorders.* Baltimore, Md.: Johns Hopkins University Press, 2003.

■ DYSTHYMIC DISORDER

See: Related Disorders

■ EATING DISORDERS AND DEPRESSION

See: Bipolar Disorder; Depression, Symptoms of; Seasonal Affective Disorder (SAD)

■ ETHNICITY AND DEPRESSION

The status of depression—a mental disorder caused by a chemical imbalance in the brain—as it pertains to members of racial and ethnic groups in the United States. Depression is one of the major mental disorders affecting ethnic groups: joblessness, poverty, and a lack of acceptable health care have conspired to make depression a significant health problem for all U.S. minorities.

In 2003, the *American Journal of Public Health* published a report, "Racial/Ethnic Differences in Rates of Depression Among Preretirement Adults," that concluded depression is more frequent among members of minority groups of color than among whites. The report also concluded that members of minority groups who suffer from depression do not receive quality mental health treatment. Compared to whites, minorities in the United States are more likely to be unemployed, have no health insurance, and have less access to mental health treatment.

In 2006, the New York State Assembly held hearings on depression and suicide among ethnic groups in New York. Lawmakers learned that teenage Hispanic girls in New York City are hospitalized for depression after attempting suicide at a rate of 388 girls per 100,000, according to figures supplied by the New York City Department of

Mental Health. Concurrently, teenage white girls are hospitalized at a rate of 374 girls per 100,000. Moreover, Asian women who are 65 and older have a suicide rate of 11.6 percent per 100,000 women. That is more than double the rate for non-Hispanic white women in that age group. Additionally, a survey of older Asians in New York City found that 40 percent had symptoms of depression.

While African Americans exhibit symptoms of depression at the same rate as the general population, they are less likely to seek help. According to writer Terri M. Williams, who authored the book *Black Pain: It Just Looks Like We're Not Hurting,* African Americans look at depression as a sign of weakness. As such, only a few seek help.

"Black people would rather say that they have a relative in jail before they will acknowledge that they have a mental illness," Williams said in an interview with *U.S. News.* "But many of my white friends and colleagues who are very much more open will tell you that they can't make an appointment because they are going to see their therapist. But it's a very different experience in the African-American community."

Researchers at Harvard School of Public Health looked at the rate of depression among blacks between 2001 and 2003. The survey found that 56.5 percent of African Americans were depressed at some time in their lives. The study also reported that 56 percent of Caribbean blacks reported bouts of depression during their lifetime. Only 38.6 percent of whites complained of being depressed. In addition, while only 45 percent of African Americans and 24.3 percent of Caribbean blacks received any form of therapy for their depression, about 57 percent of white Americans with major depression received treatment.

PROPER TREATMENT

For minorities, mental health care in the United States is not available equally. About 15 percent of the U.S. population uses some form of mental health service each year. However, studies show that whites have better access to proper treatment than minorities. Hurdles in treatment form between the races because mental health services are complex and uneven. Those who are better educated and make more money are more likely than the poor to receive proper treatment for depression and other behavioral issues.

A MELTING POT

The strength of the United States is the result of the diverse backgrounds and communities of its citizens. However, this cultural and ethnic diversity has increased the demand for proper mental health services tailored specifically to various racial and ethnic communities.

Unfortunately, poverty, different cultures, language barriers, and the lack of access to adequate health care have put most ethnic groups at a severe disadvantage compared to the rest of the population. In short, minorities are simply not getting the mental health care they need or deserve. According to the Office of Minority Health, part of the U.S. Department of Health and Human Services, the following statistics prevail:

- The suicide rate for African American men in 2005 was five times that of African American women.
- African Americans are 30 percent more likely to report having serious psychological problems than whites.
- Asian Americans have the highest suicide rate of women over age 65.
- The suicide rate for Hispanic girls in grades 9–12 in 2005 was 60 percent higher than the suicide rate for white girls in the same age group.
- The suicide rate for adolescent American Indian/Alaska natives is two to five times the rate for whites in the same age groups.

These and other statistics underscore that adequate mental health care is out of reach for many minorities. That schism was profoundly illustrated at the beginning of the new millennium by the Surgeon General of the United States.

EYE-OPENING REPORT

In 2001, the *Surgeon General's Report on Mental Health: Culture, Race, and Ethnicity* highlighted the problem that minority groups face when it comes to seeking treatment for depression and other disorders. Because minorities make up the bulk of the poor, the report was a call for action and an eye-opener for those in the mental health field.

The report concluded that poor people are at least two to three times more likely than those at the highest end of the economic ladder to experience a mental health disorder. According to the surgeon general, minorities

- have less access to mental health care;
- have less mental health care services available to them;

■ are less likely to receive needed mental health services;

■ in treatment often receive a poorer quality of mental health care; and

■ are discriminated against in the type of mental health care they receive.

While minorities are no more likely than whites to be the victims of mental illnesses, various barriers keep African Americans, Hispanics, American Indians, and Asian Americans from getting treatment. For those minorities who do get treatment, it is substandard at best.

"While mental disorders may touch all Americans, either directly or indirectly, all do not have equal access to treatment and services," U.S. Surgeon General Dr. David Satcher said at the time the report was issued. "The revolution in science," he continued, "that has led to effective treatments for mental illnesses needs to benefit every American of every race, ethnicity and culture."

"Everyone in need must have access to high-quality, effective and affordable mental health services," Satcher continued. "Too often, our mental health problems are left to play themselves out in the nation's streets, homeless centers, . . . and prisons."

DID YOU KNOW?

Feelings of Depression in African Americans

Feelings	Non-Hispanic Black	Non-Hispanic White
Sadness	3.7	2.4
Hopelessness	1.9	1.8
Worthlessness	1.3	1.8
Everything is an effort	6.8	4.5

The chart shows that a higher percentage of African Americans 18 years old or older describe feelings of "sadness," "hopelessness," or "everything is an effort all of the time" in comparison to white Americans.

Centers for Disease Control and Prevention, Summary Health Statistics for U.S. Adults: 2007.

AFRICAN AMERICANS AND MENTAL HEALTH

African Americans seem to be the minority group that suffers the most from of inadequate mental health care. The poverty rate among blacks is significantly higher than any other group. The surgeon general reported that 25 percent of African Americans do not have health insurance.

The surgeon general also reported that African Americans often postpone treatment, and when they do seek help, they usually go to hospital emergency rooms. Moreover, there are few African Americans working in the mental health field, leaving few alternatives for blacks wishing to be treated by members of their own race.

HISPANICS

Inequities in mental health care also affect the Hispanic community. Hispanic Americans are the fastest-growing minority group in the United States. They total more than 35 million people. Government statistics indicate that by 2050, the population of Hispanic Americans will increase to 97 million, roughly one-fourth of the total U.S. population.

According to the surgeon general, adult Mexicans who come to the United States have lower rates of mental illness than Mexican Americans born here. Studies also show that Hispanic children in the United States are more depressed than white children. Hispanic American children have more **anxiety**-related issues and greater behavioral problems than whites. The trend does not end when Hispanic Americans get older. One study suggests that 26 percent of older Hispanic Americans are depressed.

In addition, Hispanics living in poverty are twice as likely to report some type of psychological distress as Hispanics living above the poverty level. Hispanic men are five times more likely to commit suicide than Hispanic women. Hispanic girls in grades 9–12 are 80 times more likely to attempt suicide than white girls at the same grade level. Additionally, whites are three times more likely to receive mental health treatment than Hispanics.

Although the Hispanic population in the United States is growing, the mental health profession is lagging behind in treating this unique ethnic and cultural group. According to the surgeon general, about 37 percent of Hispanics in the United States are less likely than other minority groups to have health insurance. In addition, Hispanics who attempt to receive mental health treatment face language barriers than

DID YOU KNOW?

Feelings of Depression in Hispanic Americans

Feelings	Hispanic	Non-Hispanic White
Sadness	4.9	2.4
Hopelessness	3.1	1.8
Worthlessness	2.6	1.8
Everything is an effort	4.8	4.5

Hispanics 18 years old or older are more likely to report feelings of "sadness," "hopelessness," "worthlessness," or "everything is an effort" than whites in the United States.

Centers for Disease Control and Prevention, Summary Health Statistics for U.S. Adults, 2007.

can complicate their recovery. Most mental health providers in the United States do not speak Spanish.

Moreover, Hispanics born in the United States are more likely to suffer from a mental illness than Hispanics born in Mexico or living in Puerto Rico. Additionally, while the rate of mental illness among Hispanic Americans is the same for whites, Hispanics are more likely to suffer from depression, suicide, and anxiety disorders.

NATIVE AMERICANS

Many Native American and indigenous Alaskan groups live in rural areas where mental health treatment is limited. According to the surgeon general, Native Americans have a suicide rate that is 50 percent higher than the rest of the U.S. population.

While location plays a role in the treatment options Native Americans have, there is a more insidious influence that keeps Native Americans suffering from mental illness from seeking treatment. In most Native American societies, there is a cultural stigma associated with mental illnesses. As a result, Native Americans use mental health services at a lower rate than whites, regardless of age of gender.

In 2006, suicide was the leading cause of death for Native Americans and Alaska Natives between the ages of 10 and 34. Native Americans

DID YOU KNOW?

Feelings of Depression in Native Americans

Age	American Indian/ Alaska Native Men	Non-Hispanic White Men
15–24 years	32.7	18.4
25–44 years	29.4	26.6
45–64 years	16.8	28.2
65 years and over	NA	33.2
All ages	18.9	21.2

The chart illustrates the suicide rate in 2005 for Native American and Native Alaska males compared to the suicide rate for white males.

Centers for Disease Control and Prevention, 2008.

and Alaska Natives are three times more likely to experience feelings of sadness or hopelessness compared to whites.

WHAT TO DO

Mental health officials have proposed several recommendations to help minorities get the mental health treatment they need. These measures include increased research that is specific to minorities, making treatment more culturally and linguistically friendly, linking mental health care with primary medical care, and making sure that isolated areas of the country are covered by mental health services.

See also: Depression and Families; Gender and Depression

FURTHER READING

Keena, Kathleen. *Adolescent Depression: Outside/In.* Lincoln, Nebr.: iuniverse: 2005.

Schab, Lisa M. *Beyond the Blues: A Workbook to Help Teens Overcome Depression.* Oakland, Calif: Instant Help Books, 2008.

Zucker, Faye. *Depression.* Life Balance. New York: Scholastic, 2003.

■ GENDER AND DEPRESSION

The different ways in which males and females experience persistent unhappiness. During the past 20 years, numerous studies have shown that women are twice as likely as men to suffer from depression. This is true in every social group and at every educational level, according to a 2001 article in *Psychiatric Times.* While there is no single explanation for the disparity, many reasons have been suggested to explain why so many more women and adolescent girls get depressed than men and adolescent boys.

EXPLAINING THE GAP

Before **puberty,** girls and boys are equally likely to be depressed, with approximately 10 to 15 percent of all children showing moderate to severe signs of depression at some time during their childhood. It is only at puberty that girls start getting depressed in significantly larger numbers than boys, according to psychologist Anita Gurian of the New York University School of Medicine. This leads many researchers to suspect that female **hormones** and the **menstrual cycle** play a part in causing depression. This view is bolstered by studies that show that after **menopause,** women are no more likely than men of the same age to suffer from depression.

While estrogen, the primary female hormone, may affect emotions and moods, a specific biological mechanism explaining the role of hormones in depression has never been found. Furthermore, because most girls and women will never experience a major depression in their lives, estrogen levels cannot be the whole answer to the gender gap riddle. After all, one-third of all people who suffer from depression are male.

Everybody suffers some unhappiness sometime. Sadness, pain, heartbreak, and disappointment enter into every human existence. Depression, however, is a mental disorder characterized by a prolonged sense of desolation and hopelessness. It is natural to be sad if a relative dies, but if a person feels despairing month after month, he or she should seek medical attention. When depression strikes teenagers, it can interfere with making friends, doing well at school, and learning to be independent. Because adolescent depression can prevent or delay these important goals, it is especially important for teenagers to recognize and treat ongoing misery. Without medical intervention, periods of depression are likely to continue into adulthood.

If estrogen does not explain the gender gap, could there be other biological reasons why teenage girls are more likely than boys to suffer from depression? Some studies suggest that everyday stress affects females more than males. In females, the hypothalamic-pituitary-adrenal (HPA) hormone system is more reactive to stress, and this reaction, which involves increased production of the hormone **cortisol**, may contribute to a greater susceptibility to depression. Most researchers, however, feel that the effects of HPA hormones are minimal compared to the influence of psychological and social factors.

Psychological factors

Boys are generally happy with the changes that puberty brings. Additional muscles and a deepening voice are usually welcome signs of maturation. However, some adolescent girls may be upset by their physical changes, especially by the additional fat on their bodies, which is a normal part of becoming a woman. Suddenly, thighs are thicker and buttocks more prominent than before. Also, as their breasts develop, many girls feel awkward and self-conscious. They may feel that their breasts are too large or too small—and in either case, they have no control at all over the outcome. They may feel upset every time a boy notices them, so that even an appreciative glance makes them cringe.

Q & A

Question: I often feel tired and unhappy. I always want to sleep or nap. When I am awake, I just feel sad. Am I suffering from depression?

Answer: Because your body is undergoing rapid growth and change, you and all adolescents need more sleep than children ages eight through 10. Make sure you are getting enough sleep at night: eight to 10 hours. If your sadness persists over time, it would be helpful for you to talk about it with a trusted adult to see if you should seek further help.

Social factors

Many teenage girls have a low self-image. Research indicates that self-esteem peaks at age nine in girls, after which it often declines, when girls come to believe they are mainly valued for their appearance. They may despair that they will never look like the stylized images of models and performers produced by the media. They may feel unhappy each time they open a fashion magazine and see impossibly thin models (often in "doctored" or manipulated images) and page after page of dieting advice that is hopelessly difficult to follow. They may become **anorexic** or depressed. Obsession with weight and appearance prevents many girls from developing their talents, skills, and athletic abilities. While boys may be improving their jump shots or building computers, too many girls are looking at the mirror, feeling morose.

Furthermore, adolescent boys and girls have different ways of coping with pressure. Boys are more likely to be violent and aggressive. They may drink or take drugs or get into fights. Girls characteristically turn inward or to their friends, who can be extremely unreliable in the early teenage years. A girl can suddenly find that for no particular reason, her friends are not speaking to her, and she will desperately try to figure out why, reproaching herself and obsessively going over real and imagined conversations. Psychologist Anita Gurian writes, "In addition to low self-esteem, some adolescent girls develop certain characteristics—pessimistic thinking, a sense of having little control over life events, and proneness to excessive worrying—which place them at risk for depression. These attributes may exaggerate the effect of stressful life events or interfere with taking action to cope with them." Also, adolescent girls are more bound up with their families and more affected by family strains, especially any stress their mothers may be suffering. Even though many women today hold important positions and support their families, many girls believe they must hide how smart they are in order to be popular with boys, a belief that contributes to low self-esteem.

One additional reason why there is a higher reported depression rate among females comes from the fact that women are more likely than men to talk about unhappiness and seek treatment. Many men and boys just try to "tough it out."

BOYS AND DEPRESSION

The tendency of men and boys to ignore or deprecate their own feelings is a problem in male depression, according to a 2002 article in *Psychology Today.* If boys do not recognize their own feelings of sadness or inadequacy, they cannot communicate these feelings to a parent or another trusted adult and get help. Some depressed boys may never have learned to identify and talk about their emotions, perhaps because their fathers were hesitant to do this. It is vital for boys, like girls, to learn and express what they feel. It is especially important for boys to handle negative feelings such as anger, fear, frustration, loneliness, and doubt, because depressed boys are at special risk for causing or suffering physical damage through fighting, drinking, and other risky behavior. This "acting out" is often a sign of depression rather than aggression. As depression in boys can lead to hyperactivity, irritability, and difficulty in concentration, sometimes depressed boys are mistakenly diagnosed with ADHD.

A recent article in the *Archives of General Psychiatry* links exposure to TV to depression in young adulthood, especially in young men. The chief researcher, Dr. Brian Primack of the University of Pittsburgh School of Medicine, believes that watching handsome, successful men solving problems or selling products can make teenage boys feel insecure and inadequate by contrast. Others believe that excessive TV viewing is a symptom and not a cause of depression.

TREATMENT

The two most common ways of treating depression are medication and therapy, and a combination of the two seems to work best of all. Therapy can help people better understand themselves and find their own ways to increase happiness and stability. With a sympathetic and qualified therapist, patients can discuss their problems, feel less isolated, and work out healthy outcomes.

There are many kinds of therapy and practitioners. Recent research published in the *Journal of the American Medical Association* indicates that cognitive behavioral therapy (CBT) is especially effective in preventing and treating depression in teens. CBT does not delve into the history of the patient; rather, it teaches coping strategies and positive thinking. In a recent study, all participants had either a history of depression or at least one parent who was depressed, which put those in the study at an elevated risk for depression. Half were randomly chosen to be part of an intervention program, which consisted of eight weekly group sessions followed by six monthly sessions. The therapists taught problem-solving skills and other ways to help their adolescent patients change unrealistic and negative thinking, which is especially common in girls. Many of the patients managed to break long habits of self-blame and self-hatred. Only one in five of the treated patients experienced further depression, compared to one in three of the untreated or **control group**.

Many therapists recommend that their depressed patients use medications to achieve a happier outlook. For several decades, psychiatrists and other physicians have prescribed antidepressants for people suffering from depression. Now it seems that there may be a gender gap in how well antidepressants work, as well as in the frequency of depression itself. Dr. Susan Kornstein, head of the outpatient psychiatry clinic at the Virginia Commonwealth University, has recently reported that women respond better than men to certain drugs, such as sertraline. Sertraline is a serotonin reuptake inhibitor, or SSRI drug. This means it makes more **serotonin** available to the brain, and serotonin is involved in controlling mood, sleep, appetite, and other functions that are affected by depression. Dr. Kornstein also found that men respond better than women to imipramine, an older antidepressant.

As most antidepressants cause some negative side effects, people often turn to natural ways to overcome depression. Because physical activity has long been known to ease depression, counselors will often recommend that their depressed students take up a sport. This can be especially helpful for girls who were not previously physically active. Mastering any new activity can help people feel they can get their lives back in control. Furthermore, physical exercise results in the production of serotonin and endorphins. Endorphins are compounds produced by glands at the base of the brain during strenuous exercise. "Runner's high" is thought to be linked to the production of endorphins; exercise can make people feel very good. However, it is often hard to motivate people suffering from depression to do what might make them feel better. A mother might recommend that her depressed daughter go for a run, while the girl just wants to crawl into bed.

Fact Or Fiction?

Eating the right foods can help your mood.

The Facts: Sometimes carbohydrates, such as pasta or bread, can provide a temporary lift in your spirits, but if you are deeply unhappy over the course of several weeks you may want to consider therapeutic options. Eating well and maintaining a healthy weight can help stave off depression in girls. However, plenty of thin people are depressed, so diet is one of the many factors that may affect depression.

A few researchers believe that proper diet can be beneficial. Omega-three fatty acids, found in some fish, may help raise a person's outlook. A diet that includes salmon and other fatty fish may improve mood in both girls and boys. Another approach is to increase carbohydrate consumption. Some people just crave carbs, and when they eat a high-carb meal, they feel better in about 20 minutes. However, it is most important to eat a balanced diet that includes plenty of fresh vegetables, fruit, and protein.

The important thing to remember is that depression can be treated. With treatment, most people who suffer from depression can learn how to live happy and productive lives.

FURTHER READING

Gurian, Anita, Ph.D. "Depression in Adolescence: Does Gender Matter?" Available online. URL: www.aboutourkids.org. Accessed March 23, 2010.

Mayo Clinic Staff. "Depression in Women: Understanding the Gender Gap," Available online. URL: www.mayoclinic.com/health/depression. Accessed March 23, 2010.

■ GENETICS OF MOOD AND ANXIETY DISORDERS

The role of genetics, or inherited characteristics, in mental illness. Researchers have conducted many studies of families and twins that show mental disorders tend to run in families. For example, a close relative of someone who suffers from depression is twice as likely to suffer from depression as someone who does not have a depressed relative. However, it is generally thought that mood and anxiety disorders cannot be directly traced to individual **genes.** Rather, many scientists say that alleles (or variants) of some genes, on different **chromosomes,** work together to make it more likely for certain individuals to become mentally ill. Just because someone might inherit these genes does not mean they will become mentally ill. Instead, a person's genetic makeup might **predispose** that person to a mental disorder.

THE ROLE OF ENVIRONMENT

The environment in which a person lives is an important factor in mental illness. This is good news, because we can change our environment—such as changing schools—more easily than we can change our genes.

Luckily, no one is fated to become mentally ill, and once ill, no one is fated to stay that way. A person might have the "wrong genes" and never know it because he or she lives a happy, fulfilled life. Even those without any genetic predisposition to a mental disorder can become depressed when bad things happen to them, such as the loss of a parent or friend.

Jordan Smoller, M.D., director of the Psychiatric Genetics Program in Mood and Anxiety Disorders at Massachusetts General Hospital (MGH), is one of the nation's leading researchers into the genetics of mental disorders. According to Dr. Smoller, . . . "genes act essentially like risk factors, like cholesterol is a risk factor for heart disease." Many factors, from upbringing and environment to stressful situations, work together, along with genetics, to determine whether someone will experience a mood or anxiety disorder—or, more likely, both.

Q & A

Question: When my mother gets angry with me, she says, "You have the crazy gene, just like your father." It's true that I look like my dad, and sometimes he has periods of major depression. Will I get this, too?

Answer: Your mother is wrong. There is no such thing as a "crazy gene." Rather, dozens of genes might make it somewhat more likely for you to be depressed than for someone without a depressed parent. Statistics show that not all children of depressed parents become depressed themselves.

The fact that your father is, at times, depressed is an unhappy circumstance in your life—an environmental factor as well as a genetic one—but this does not mean you will be depressed. However, you should be especially alert to symptoms of depression and speak to a trusted adult if you feel unhappy for weeks at a time.

GENETIC STUDIES CONTRIBUTE TO A NEW FINDING
For decades, mood and anxiety disorders were considered distinct and unrelated problems. However, according to an article in January

2002 in the *American Journal of Psychiatry,* patients with major depression invariably exhibit symptoms of anxiety, and more than 90 percent of patients with panic disorder (an anxiety disorder) also have a mood disorder. (In the same patient, one type of disorder usually predominates, causing much more distress.) Drugs that are effective in one area are also effective in the other. Therefore, researchers and doctors now believe that mood and anxiety disorders are often **comorbid**. In other words, these disorders may occur together.

Genetics studies support the theory of comorbidity. According to an article in *Psychological Medicine* in May 2005, "Twin studies show that comorbidity . . . between anxiety disorders and depression is explained by a shared genetic vulnerability for both disorders." It appears that variants of certain **neurotransmitter** genes are contributing factors to both mood and anxiety disorders. (A neurotransmitter sends nerve impulses across a synapse—or gap—to another nerve, muscle, or gland.)

In June 2009, researchers at the University of Pennsylvania found a genetic link between anxiety, depression, and **insomnia**. Scientists looked at information from hundreds of twins to reach this conclusion. Still, even if one identical twin suffered from insomnia, the other twin did not necessarily have trouble falling asleep. Rather, the second twin was more likely to suffer from insomnia than if he or she were a fraternal twin, who is less closely related. Since identical twins have identical genes, environmental factors must also contribute to insomnia, as they do to anxiety and depression.

AN OPEN QUESTION

An article in the August 2008 issue of *Behavioral Neuroscience* also supports the idea of a genetic element in mental illness. Scientists from the University of Bonn, Germany, even named an individual gene that they believe may play a role in anxiety disorders—the COMT gene. People who carry a common variant (Met-158) of the COMT gene have a much larger "startle reflex" than those who have the other variant (Val-158). The startle reflex is measured by attaching electrodes to the eye muscles that cause a person to blink, which people do when emotionally aroused. Both genetic groups were shown disturbing pictures, and the people with the Met-158 variant blinked more intensely than the Val-158 group. It is believed that a strong startle reflex makes it easier for a person to feel anxious. Met-158 carriers seem more deeply affected by unpleasant images than the other group and less able to shake them.

Researchers, who are constantly evaluating the link between genes and mental disorders, vary in their conclusions. For example, in June 2009, researchers writing in the *Journal of the American Medical Association* argued that there is actually no genetic predisposition for depression. They dismissed studies that claim to have found a genetic basis for depression because these studies have not been, or cannot be, duplicated. Duplication is the gold standard for scientific research because it validates the conclusions of the original study. According to this study, "few disorders have proven as resistant to gene identification as psychiatric illnesses."

THE GENETICS OF MEDICATION

One use of genetics in treating mental disorders is to establish what drugs might help individuals. This personalized medicine is known as **pharmacogenetics.** It is especially important in the field of mental illness because different **psychoactive** drugs affect people in different ways, and it can take several weeks for a drug to have an effect. A patient does not want to wait weeks to find out that the drug he or she is taking will not work, or that it causes uncomfortable side effects. New tests involving genetic variations in liver enzymes are starting to predict how a person will react to certain drugs. (These tests are an outgrowth of the **Human Genome Project.**) Liver enzyme tests can help doctors prescribe the right medication at the right dosage the first time, without trial and error. Knowing ahead of time which medicines are likely to work would be a major breakthrough in human health. Soon, genetics may even tell us which individuals will respond as well to a **placebo** as to a pharmaceutically active drug. This is valuable information, because a placebo is less likely to produce unpleasant side effects.

Fact Or Fiction?

Curing a mental disorder is just a matter of taking the right drug.

The Facts: While the right pharmaceutical can make a big difference in one's treatment, almost every study indicates that counseling is an important component for achieving a full and lasting recovery. Talking about one's symptoms and problems with a trusted and well trained health professional is an important part of a complete treatment plan.

FURTHER READING

Mattis, Sara G., Thomas H. Ollendick, and Martin Herbert. *Panic Disorder and Anxiety in Adolescence.* Oxford, U.K.: Blackwell Publishers, 2002.

Moorman, Margaret. *My Sister's Keeper: Learning to Cope with a Sibling's Mental Illness.* New York: W. W. Norton, 2002.

▮ GRIEVING

See: Related Disorders

▮ MEDIA AND ANXIETY AND DEPRESSION, THE

Media or **mass media** are terms used to describe the various methods of mass communication, such as television, radio, magazines, newspapers, and the Internet. Most people, including children, are exposed to the media every day. According to a 1999 Kaiser Family Foundation study called "Kids & Media at the New Millennium" study, most children spend at least part of their day with more than one media at a time. They might read a magazine while watching television or listening to the radio. Young people ages eight to 18 spend an average of 6¾ hours a day with various forms of the media. In fact, only 5 percent of all children spend an hour or less a day exposed to media.

In the past, families, religious institutions, schools, and community leaders were responsible for teaching cultural values. Values are the fundamental beliefs of an individual or a group of people. **Cultural values** determine what standards, behaviors, or attitudes will be encouraged in a society. George Gerbner, a researcher who has spent 30 years monitoring the cultural impact of television, says the mass media has taken over the role of instilling cultural values. The mass media's role in instilling cultural values raises important questions. The way mental disorders or any other illnesses are portrayed can have a serious impact on how people with those disorders are perceived. For example, if negative images of people with depression predominate in the media, the general public is likely to hold more negative views of people with depression.

STEREOTYPES

A stereotype is a judgment about an individual based on the characteristics of a group. It reduces individuals to categories or labels by denying an individual's unique qualities. When you watch television, surf the Web, or read magazines, you often see people portrayed in stereotypical ways. You may see people with mental illnesses acting "crazy" or they may be shown as dangerous or unpredictable. Because these images are so negative, you and others may find yourself feeling uncomfortable around people who suffer from mental disorders, without knowing why. These negative stereotypes may result not only in discrimination in housing, education, and employment but also in social isolation.

According to George Gerbner, television characters with mental disorders are four times more likely to be violent than other characters. Otto Wahl of George Mason University uncovered similar patterns in films. He found that between 1985 and 1995, Hollywood released more than 150 films that included characters with mental illnesses. The majority of them were murderers and other villains.

Media images in programming intended for young children also contain negative stereotypes. In *Good Burger,* a film based on the Nickelodeon series *Keenan and Kel,* the characters visit a place called Demented Hills Asylum, where psychiatric patients in straitjackets eat cards and growl menacingly at visitors. Such images could easily give young children the impression that people who have mental disorders are less than human.

DID YOU KNOW?

Kids' Choice of Media

Children eight and older are nearly three times as likely to choose computers over television if forced to pick one form of media to have with them on a desert island (33 percent chose a computer; only 13 percent chose a television).

Source: Kaiser Family Foundation, November, 1999.

STIGMA

Stigma refers to the shame and disapproval attached to anything regarded as socially unacceptable. Because of the negative images and stereotypes portrayed in the media, people who experience depression may believe they should be ashamed of their condition. They may feel even more isolated. In fact, many people with mental health problems don't seek treatment because they are embarrassed by what others may think of them. This can be dangerous and even life threatening. According to the National Institute of Mental Health, about 60 percent of those who commit suicide in a given year have had a mental disorder such as depression. So treatment is essential. The stigma attached to mental disorders based on media images may prevent sufferers from getting help.

Images in the media may lead some people to think that people who are depressed are weak-willed or are not willing to try hard enough to feel better.

Recently the media has tried to portray people with mental disorders more realistically. Well-known celebrities, such as actress Brooke Shields, musician Billy Joel, and comedian Jim Carey all have suffered from depression. Each has been very open about his or her condition, reducing some of the stigma surrounding depression.

TEENS SPEAK

I Was Too Embarrassed to Get Help

After my parents went to bed at night, I'd go to the family room and turn on the TV. If I kept the volume really low, I could stay there until I heard their alarm clock in the morning and they'd never know. I hadn't slept at night for four or five months. I would sleep when I got home from school and get up just in time for dinner.

I didn't know why I couldn't sleep. When I went to bed at night, I couldn't stop thoughts from zooming through my head and it felt terrible. Staying awake and secretly watching television was the best solution I could find to keep my mind quiet.

I was also crying all the time—not around people, but I stayed away from people as much as I could. I'd cry at ads on TV, I'd cry listening to a song on the radio, or I'd cry because I couldn't find my hairbrush or something like that. It was really bad.

One late night, I was watching a celebrity news show. The reporter said Janet Jackson had spoken to *Newsweek* magazine about her experiences with depression. At that time in my life, Janet was my idol. I had all her albums, and I thought I knew her life story. It turns out she suffered from depression for two years. She told reporters about it and talked about how she was feeling better after being treated for the depression. I don't know why, but I felt less alone. I felt like I wasn't the only one who was having trouble.

When the show went to a commercial, they had an ad for what to do if you were suffering from depression. Somehow, I found the courage to call the 800 number. I spoke to a really nice man who gave me the phone numbers of people I could talk to where I lived. He definitely didn't think I was crazy, but he thought it would be good for me to talk with a professional.

After I started talking with the school therapist, things started getting better. Sometimes I think that if I hadn't seen Janet Jackson dealing with her depression, I might still be crying all the time and never sleeping.

MOVING TOWARD A FAIR REPRESENTATION

Until recently, the media portrayed people with depression as crazy, dangerous, even animalistic. While many images are still misleading and negative, people in the public eye are speaking out about their own mental disorders. Slowly, the media is beginning to treat people with mental disorders more respectfully. Realistic and balanced coverage of mental disorders may make it easier for people with mental disorders to get the professional help they need.

See also: Morbidity and Mortality

FURTHER READING

Pettit, Jeremy W. *The Interpersonal Solution to Depression: A Workbook for Changing How You Feel by Changing How You Relate.* New Harbinger Self-Help Workbook. Oakland, Calif.: New Harbinger Publications, 2005.

■ MEDICATION

See: Treatment of Anxiety Disorders; Treatment of Depression

■ MENTAL HEALTH PROFESSIONALS, TYPES OF

Specially trained individuals who treat patients with behavioral, mental, and emotional disorders. Mental health professionals include psychiatrists, psychologists, social workers, and counselors, among others. Each professional has specific areas of expertise. Some psychiatrists and psychologists, for example, treat only children, while some counselors work with those suffering from drug and alcohol addiction.

According to the U.S. Surgeon General, about 15 percent of adults in the United States use some form of mental health service in a given year, and one in five people suffer from some form of mental illness. Many receive treatment through health care providers, social service agencies, local clergy, or school systems.

Treating the mentally ill is costly. The U.S. Surgeon General estimates that the indirect cost of helping people cope with depression in the United States is $80 billion a year.

MISUNDERSTOOD MALADY

For thousands of years, those suffering from mental disorders could not receive treatment because they were misunderstood. Society shunned and stigmatized those suffering from any mental illness. In the 1600s, the "insane" or "mad" were often accused of being witches or possessed by a demon. With time, some treatment was available, but it was haphazard at best. Those deemed "mad" were often locked away from society in asylums. In these institutions, patients would undergo sometimes barbaric treatments to "cure" them of their affliction.

Within the last 30 or 40 years, there has been a revolution in science that has expanded our understanding of mental illness and improved mental health care. Depression, eating disorders, bipolar disorder, anxiety disorders, attention-deficit-hyperactivity disorder, and other mental disorders are now treatable, thanks to better therapies and medications. Early diagnosis and treatment have improved the quality of life for millions.

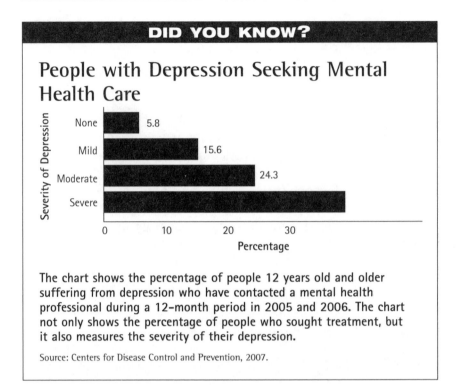

DID YOU KNOW?

People with Depression Seeking Mental Health Care

Severity of Depression

- None: 5.8
- Mild: 15.6
- Moderate: 24.3
- Severe

Percentage (0, 10, 20, 30)

The chart shows the percentage of people 12 years old and older suffering from depression who have contacted a mental health professional during a 12-month period in 2005 and 2006. The chart not only shows the percentage of people who sought treatment, but it also measures the severity of their depression.

Source: Centers for Disease Control and Prevention, 2007.

PSYCHOTHERAPY

One of the ways to treat those suffering from mental disorders such as depression is through the process of psychotherapy. Psychotherapy is a general term used by health professionals to describe "talk therapy."

During psychotherapy, a person learns about his or her problems, feelings, thoughts, and behaviors by talking with a professional counselor or therapist. As patients talk, they can gain insight and knowledge about their condition. Therapy also can provide a patient with numerous coping mechanisms, such as stress relief. Psychotherapy treatment plans can last a few months or several years, depending on the severity of a person's illness. Through psychotherapy, patients can explore such problems as grief, anger, relationship stress, work conflicts, school performance, and sleep disorders, among other things.

Generally speaking, psychotherapy poses little risk. However, patients might feel uncomfortable exploring various situations, such as physical or sexual abuse or even fear of the dark. By talking through these problems, patients can learn to manage anxiety and stress.

HELPERS ALL

On the front line of treating mental disorders such as anxiety and depression are a myriad of mental health professionals. They include the following:

- **psychiatrist:** A psychiatrist is a medical doctor who specializes in the diagnosis and treatment of mental illnesses. Because psychiatrists are physicians, they can prescribe medication. A psychiatrist must have a state license and should be certified or eligible for certification by the American Board of Psychiatry and Neurology.

- **child/adolescent psychiatrist:** This is a specialized psychiatrist who treats emotional and behavioral problems in children and adolescents. Child/adolescent psychiatrists are qualified to prescribe medication.

- **psychologist:** Most psychologists have a Ph.D., an advanced educational degree, in psychology from an

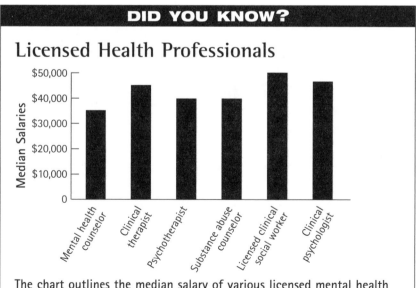

DID YOU KNOW?

Licensed Health Professionals

The chart outlines the median salary of various licensed mental health counselors. These professionals all undergo specific training to help people needing treatment.

Source: Adapted from Payscale.com, 2009.

accredited university and have completed an internship under the supervision of an experienced psychologist. Many psychologists are qualified to treat people individually or in group settings. They are not trained in the practice of medicine and do not receive medical licenses for prescribing drugs.

- **clinical social worker:** A clinical social worker or clinical therapist is required to have a master's degree in social work. Like psychologists, clinical social workers are trained to diagnose and treat individuals in a one-on-one setting or in a group. Clinical social workers can assist patients in dealing with state or government agencies. They are sometimes called on to serve as case managers for those trying to navigate the mental health system.

- **licensed professional counselor:** This mental health provider is required to have a master's degree in psychology, counseling, or a related field.

- **mental health counselor:** Mental health counselors are required to hold a master's degree and have several years of supervised clinical work experience. They are trained to diagnose and provide individual and group counseling.

- **certified alcohol and drug abuse counselor:** These substance abuse counselors are specifically trained to help those who abuse alcohol or drugs.

- **nurse psychotherapist:** A nurse psychotherapist is a registered nurse trained in psychiatric and mental health nursing.

- **marital and family therapist:** These counselors help couples and families work through various emotional and behavioral situations.

- **pastoral counselor:** Some members of the clergy have special training to help people with emotional and behavioral problems.

- **sex therapist:** A sex therapist is trained to help people deal with their concerns about sexual function and feelings that affect a person's sex life.

Fact Or Fiction?

Clinical social workers can prescribe medication.

The Facts: Clinical social workers, along with many other mental health professionals, are not allowed to prescribe medications. Only psychiatrists and some nurses who specialize in psychiatry and mental health can write a prescription.

MAKING THE CALL

Seeking treatment for a mental disorder is not easy, but it could be the most important thing you ever do. Finding the right therapist for your condition is important. It is a good idea to first describe your symptoms to a family doctor, a school counselor, a family member, or a member of the clergy. They can often suggest what type of mental health professional you should see.

Once you have settled on a therapist, spend a few minutes on the phone with that person asking about how he or she works with patients and his or her philosophy regarding the treatment of mental disorders such as yours. In addition, ask the therapist if he or she has a specialty. Some counselors work with teens on any problem, while others focus on alcohol and drug addiction. If you feel comfortable with the counselor, make an appointment.

Fact Or Fiction?

A therapist can tell my mom and dad what we talked about in therapy.

The Facts: Do not worry. Ethically, all mental health professionals cannot tell anyone what you discussed in therapy. However, a therapist must by law report if someone is about to harm another person or her/himself.

Once you begin treatment, there might be a time when you won't feel comfortable with your counselor or therapist. If this is the case, do not worry. Talk about your feelings with the therapist. You also can make an appointment with a new counselor to help you overcome your problems. Being comfortable with a therapist is very important to successful in treatment.

See also: Depression and Families; Psychotherapies, Kinds of; Treatment of Anxiety Disorders; Treatment of Mood Disorders

FURTHER READING

Roberts, Michael C., and Ric G. Steel. *Handbook of Mental Health Services for Children, Adolescents, and Families.* Issues in Clinical Child Psychology. New York: Kluwer Academic/Plenum Publishers, 2005.

Brent, David, and DeQuincy Lezine. *Eight Stories Up: An Adolescent Chooses Hope Over Suicide.* Adolescent Mental Health Initiative. New York: Oxford University Press, 2008.

■ MOOD DISORDERS

See: Genetics of Mood and Anxiety Disorders; Related Disorders

■ MORBIDITY AND MORTALITY

The term *morbidity* describes the harmful effects of a disease in a population, *mortality* refers to the death rate in a given population as a result of a disorder. If mental disorders such as anxiety and depression are left untreated, they can be dangerous, even fatal.

INJURY AND ILLNESS RELATED TO DEPRESSION AND ANXIETY

Many illnesses are connected with both anxiety and depression. Some occur because of depression or an anxiety disorder, while others can cause these disorders.

More than 50 medical conditions can contribute to depression and anxiety disorders. Examples include **diabetes, hypoglycemia,** and inner ear disturbances. A relatively harmless heart condition called **mitral valve prolapse** can be another **trigger.** Thyroid problems are commonly associated with depression. Heart troubles may also contribute to mental disorders. In fact, 30 percent of people who are hospitalized for **coronary artery disease,** an obstruction in the arteries leading to the heart, experience some depression. Harvard University researchers report that about 50 percent of patients who survived a heart attack become depressed. In addition, those who became depressed after suffering a heart attack were two to three times more likely to have another heart attack compared with those who were not depressed. Researchers in the Netherlands found that one out of three people who developed depression for the first time after a heart attack died of another heart attack or stroke far more frequently than those who were not depressed after their first heart attack.

Anxiety or depression can have a negative impact on some medical conditions, including asthma and **Tourette syndrome.** The Tourette Syndrome Association defines the syndrome as an inherited, neurological disorder characterized by repeated and involuntary body movements (tics) and uncontrollable vocal sounds.

CAUSES OF DEATH

If depression and anxiety disorders are left untreated, or if there are additional complications, both can be deadly. Each has been linked to substance abuse–related fatalities, suicide, and other deadly medical conditions.

Medical causes

Some deaths among people with depression or anxiety disorders are caused by the illnesses associated with the disorders rather than the disorders themselves. For example, depression and anxiety disorders may affect heart rhythms, increase blood pressure, and alter blood clotting. They can also lead to elevated insulin and cholesterol levels. As a result, some people die from heart diseases that have been aggravated by depression.

Furthermore, depression or anxiety may result in high levels of stress hormones, such as **cortisol** and **adrenaline.** These high levels signal the body's **fight-or-flight response.** As a result, the body's healing energies may be diverted from the type of tissue repair needed to reverse heart disease.

Depression may also make it harder for patients to take the medications they need and carry out the treatments their physicians recommend. In fact, NIMH (2001) reported that heart patients who were depressed were four times as likely to die within six months as those who were not depressed. NIMH also noted that while about one in 20 American adults experiences major depression in a given year, the rate jumps to about one in three for people who have survived a heart attack.

Suicide

People suffering from depression are more likely to commit suicide than other people. NIMH (2003) reported that more than 90 percent of those who commit suicide have depression or another diagnosable mental or substance abuse disorder.

Q & A

Question: If I tell an adult that my friend is depressed, won't I be betraying a trust?

Answer: Depression, which saps energy and self-esteem, interferes with a person's ability to seek help. Many parents may not understand the seriousness of depression or of thoughts of death or suicide. It is an act of friendship to share your concerns with a trusted adult.

Depression does not have to lead to suicide. In fact, most people who are depressed do not attempt to take their own lives. According to the National Alliance for the Mentally Ill (2003), approximately 80 to 90 percent of people who suffer from depression can be treated. Treating disorders such as depression and substance abuse is essential in reducing the likelihood of suicide. Like depression, suicide is preventable. No one is a "lost cause."

Substance abuse

Many of the deaths associated with depression and anxiety disorders are from the effects of substance abuse. An example is **cirrhosis** of the liver, which often occurs among people with alcohol and other substance abuse problems, which in turn are also related to depression and anxiety.

People suffering from mental disorders may try to "drown their sorrows" with drugs or alcohol. According to research reported by the National Center for Health Statistics (2002), the top three causes of death for 15- to 24-year-olds are automobile crashes, homicide, and suicide. Alcohol is a leading factor in all three causes of death.

Many people suffering from anxiety and depression behave recklessly and put themselves in serious danger after using drugs or alcohol.

RATES

The World Health Organization (1996) released an international study indicating that anxiety and depression are the disorders most likely to appear simultaneously. A disorder is said to be **comorbid** if it happens in conjunction with another. In many cases, those suffering from anxiety disorders also suffer from depression.

Depression is a risk factor in determining the likelihood of suicide. The R. Samuel McLaughlin Addiction and Mental Health Information Centre (2003) reported that 15 percent of people who have significant depression commit suicide. However, the Mayo Clinic suggests that the suicide rate for patients with depression is 2 to 9 percent. In addition, the American Psychiatric Association (APA) reported that 53 percent of young people who commit suicide abuse substances.

According to a 2002 article by Dr. William R. Yates of the University of Oklahoma at Tulsa Health Sciences Center, anxiety disorders may lead to suicide with or without comorbid mental disorders such as depression. Yates noted that anxiety disorders have high rates of comorbidity with depression and substance abuse. Some of the increased risk of death associated with anxiety disorders may be related to this high rate of comorbidity. He also reported there may be an increased risk for **cardiovascular** (relating to the heart and blood vessels) diseases and fatalities in those people suffering with anxiety disorders.

Depression is one of the strongest risk factors in attempted suicides. Up to 90 percent of adolescents who complete suicide have a diagnosable mental disorder at the time of their death. Every day, 86 Americans kill themselves (more than 30,000 per year)—that's approximately one person every 17 minutes.

Over the last several decades, the suicide rate among young people has increased dramatically. The U.S. Surgeon General published *A Call to Action* (1999), which reported from 1952 to 1996, the incidence of suicide among adolescents and young adults nearly tripled. Since 1993, there has been a general decline in youth suicides. From 1980 to 1996, the U.S. Surgeon General (1999) reported, the rate of suicide among people ages 15 to 19 increased by 14 percent (to 9.7 per

100,000) and among persons ages 10 to 14 by 100 percent (to 1.6 deaths per 100,000). In 2002 and again in 2006, the National Vital Statistics System reported that among 10- to 24-year-old Americans, suicide was the third leading cause of death.

There are gender differences in suicide rates. The National Centers for Injury Prevention and Control (2005) reported that four times as many men as women commit suicide, but women attempt suicide three times more frequently than men.

The National Alliance for the Mentally Ill (NAMI) reported that senior citizens are at risk for fatalities related to depression. NAMI also reported that depression is the single most significant risk factor for suicide in older Americans. In addition, according to NIMH, the highest suicide rates in the United States are found among white men over age 85.

DEPRESSION AND ANXIETY DISORDERS ARE SERIOUS

Depression and anxiety disorders are more than just feeling sad or nervous. They are mental disorders that can be fatal. The good news is that treatments for both kinds of disorders have high rates of success. If you or someone you know is suffering from symptoms that may be a depression or anxiety disorder, seeking professional help is essential.

See also: Anxiety Disorders; Depression, Causes of; Risk Factors for Depression; Suicide and Depression

FURTHER READING

"Morbidity and Mortality Weekly Report." Centers for Disease Control and Prevention. http://www.cdc.gov/mmwr/.

■ OBSESSIVE-COMPULSIVE BEHAVIOR

See: Anxiety Disorders, Symptoms of

■ PANIC ATTACKS

See: Anxiety Disorders, Types of

■ PHOBIAS

Persistent, irrational fears of specific situations, activities, or objects. Phobias are anxiety disorders. They are perhaps one of the easiest mental disorders for the general public to understand, because phobias are usually exaggerations of fears almost everyone has. Phobias affect people from all walks of life, all ethnicities, and both genders. According to a British Broadcasting Corporation (BBC) report, "What Happens When Fear Turns to Phobia?," more than 10 percent of the population suffer from an extreme phobia at some point in life.

Phobias affect people of all ages. Children are most likely to experience mild phobias that go away over a relatively short period of time. The National Institute of Mental Health (NIMH) says that 11.5 million adult Americans ages 18 to 54 experience phobias in any given year. Phobias usually begin in the mid-teens. Only a few of these phobias are long lasting and disruptive to a person's lives.

Everyone suffers from fears. The difference between a fear and a phobia is that people with phobias alter their lives to avoid the situation, activity, or object they find frightening. For example, **agoraphobia** is the fear of open spaces; it literally means "fear of the marketplace." It is rational to fear an open space during a hailstorm. However, it is irrational to fear an open field on a sunny day. For someone with agoraphobia, just thinking about an open space may cause a **panic attack.** A panic attack is a period of extreme and overwhelming anxiety accompanied by physical symptoms such as palpitations (unusually deep or rapid breathing that often leads to faintness), sweating, shakiness, nausea, and dizziness, or abdominal cramps.

SYMPTOMS

For people with phobias, just thinking about whatever they fear is enough to bring on an array of physical symptoms. These emotional and physical symptoms include the following:

- feelings of panic, dread, horror, or terror
- recognition that the fear is more than the actual threat of danger deserves
- automatic and uncontrollable reactions
- rapid heartbeat, shortness of breath, trembling
- an overwhelming desire to run away

■ extreme measures taken to avoid the feared object or situation

Whenever a phobia interferes with the ability to work, socialize, or fulfill daily responsibilities, one should consult a professional for advice and treatment.

COMMON TYPES OF PHOBIA

There are three basic types of phobia:

1. **agoraphobia**: Agoraphobia is not only a fear of open spaces but also of being in a crowd, being alone in a house, and traveling alone.

2. **social anxiety disorder** or social phobia: A fear of specific or general social situations, such as meeting new people, attending gatherings, and talking to people in authority.

3. **specific phobia**: Fear of specific situations and objects, such as flying, heights, blood, thunderstorms, dogs, mice, or spiders.

DID YOU KNOW?

From Germs to Worms

A-Z of Phobia

ailurophobia: cats	alektorophobia: chickens
apiphobia: bees	arachnophobia: spiders
bacteriophobia: bacteria	bactrachophobia: reptiles
cnidophobia: stings	cynophobia: dogs
entomophobia: insects	equinophobia: horses
helminthophobia: worms	ichthyophobia: fish
mottephobia: moths	musophobia: mice
ophidiophobia: snakes	ornithophobia: birds
parasitophobia: parasites	pediculophobia: lice
pteronophobia: feathers	rodentophobia: rodents
spermophobia: germs	spheksophobia: wasps
zoophobia: animals	

Source: Phobialist.com

AGORAPHOBIA

Agoraphobia is an extreme fear of open spaces or public places. People with agoraphobia fear grocery stores, malls, other people's houses, concert halls, school, sports arenas, and just about any place but their own homes.

Typically, the sufferer fears a panic attack in a place where escape might be difficult or embarrassing. People with agoraphobia also fear being alone in any situation where escape might be difficult or help would be unavailable if needed.

Most people develop agoraphobia after suffering from one or more panic attacks. A panic attack consists of a period of intense, overwhelming terror accompanied by symptoms such as sweating, shortness of breath, or faintness. These attacks seem to occur randomly and without warning, making it impossible to predict what situation may trigger another reaction. The unpredictability of the panic attacks "trains" people to anticipate future attacks and, therefore, to fear any situation in which an attack may occur. As a result, they avoid any place or situation associated with previous panic attacks.

Agoraphobia can keep people from performing many routine tasks such as taking a bus to school or work, shopping, or visiting friends. Some people with agoraphobia become so disabled they literally will not leave their homes. If they do go out, they do so only with great distress or when accompanied by a friend or family member.

According to NIMH (2005), approximately 1.8 million American adults ages 18 and over have agoraphobia. The *Harvard's Women's Health Watch* in August 2000 reported that women are three times more likely to be diagnosed with agoraphobia than men. The American Psychiatric Association (APA) reported that two-thirds of those diagnosed with agoraphobia are women (1999). The onset of symptoms—whether sudden or gradual—usually occurs between the ages of 18 and 35.

Fact Or Fiction?

There's no such thing as social phobia. Everyone gets nervous sometimes.

The Facts: Social phobia is a real illness that can be treated with medication and therapy. Although many people are a little nervous before meeting strangers or speaking publicly, those with social phobia are excessively worried about embarrassing themselves in front of others.

SOCIAL PHOBIA

People with social anxiety disorder, or social phobia, have an overwhelming and disabling fear of embarrassment or humiliation in social situations. The Anxiety Disorders Association of America (ADAA) and NIMH report 15 million Americans suffer from this mental disorder.

People with social phobia may have difficulty speaking, eating, or even writing in front of others. As a result of these fears, many avoid activities that could, under normal circumstances, be pleasant and enjoyable. If they do participate in these activities, they experience physical symptoms of anxiety such as blushing, palpitations, or shaking.

Those who suffer from social phobia may avoid the social situations they fear or endure them with great anxiety. Sometimes people with social phobia use alcohol or other substances to try to reduce their anxiety. Although many people are nervous in social situations, those with a social phobia find them almost unbearable.

Fear of public speaking

According to the ADAA, public speaking is one of the most common types of social phobia. It is a fear of embarrassment and humiliation when speaking in front of an audience. It is a phobia that can hamper success in school or work. In many classes and work situations, it is necessary to speak publicly. A teacher calls on students to answer questions and give reports. Therapy can help most people who suffer from social phobia.

Childhood and adolescent onset

Social phobia tends to begin in childhood or adolescence. Approximately 40 percent of social phobias occur before age 10 and about 95 percent before age 20, according to the Anxiety Disorders Association of Victoria. For a child to be diagnosed with a social phobia, symptoms must persist for at least six months.

Social scientists examine the personality traits of children and teenagers in considering the frequency of social phobias among them. A report in the *American Journal of Psychiatry* suggested a connection between social phobia and behavioral inhibition, a tendency to react negatively to new situations or things.

Some infants and children are generally happy and curious about new people and things. However, a 2003 study from the Royal College of Physicians of Canada noted that roughly 15 percent are shy, withdrawn, and irritable when they are in a new situation or among new people. Often these children are irritable as infants, shy and fearful as toddlers, and quiet and introverted at school age. They are at risk of developing social phobia later in childhood or adolescence. For a child who is not fearful and participates readily in social situations, there is only a 4 to 5 percent chance he or she will develop a social phobia as a teenager. However a 1998 report published in the *American Academy of Childhood Adolescent Psychiatry* noted that if a child is fearful and avoids social situations, the chances of developing a social phobia as a teen is about 20 to 25 percent.

According to the Anxiety Disorders Association of America, the following may be symptoms of social phobia in young children:

- fear of at least one social situation (such as recess) or performance situation (such as taking a test)
- apparent fear when dealing with peers as well as when interacting with adults
- anxiety symptoms, including sweating, racing heart, stomachache, dizziness, crying, and tantrums, when faced with a feared situation
- avoidance or intense dread of feared situations
- interference with school performance or attendance, the ability to socialize with peers, or developing and maintaining relationships

Prevalence

According to the NIMH, approximately 5.3 million American adults ages 18 to 54, or about 3.7 percent of people in this age group in a given year, experience social phobia. The NIMH also reported that social phobia affects men and women in equal numbers. Often the illness lasts a lifetime, although it may become less severe or completely disappear with treatment.

SPECIFIC PHOBIAS

As the name suggestions, specific phobias are irrational fears of specific objects or situations. Exposure to the object or situation, either in real life or through one's thoughts, can cause anxiety. The *Diagnostic and Statistical Manual of Mental Disorders, Fourth Edition,* Text Revision (2000), or *DSM-IV-TR,* the main diagnostic reference of mental health professionals in the United States, once referred to "specific phobia" as "simple phobia" (American Psychiatric Association).

People with specific phobia experience an extreme, disabling, and irrational fear of something that poses little or no actual danger. The fear may cause someone to limit his or her life unnecessarily. People can develop phobic reactions to insects like spiders, activities like getting on an airplane, or social situations like eating in public.

The U.S. Surgeon General (1999) reported that approximately 8 percent of the adult population suffers from one or more specific phobias each year. According to the *DSM-IV* (2001), many specific phobias begin in childhood, with a second "peak" of onset in the mid-20s. The Ohio State University Anxiety and Stress Disorders Clinic identifies the typical age of onset for three major subsets of specific phobia.

- Natural Environment Type (example: fear of storms) phobias tend to begin primarily in childhood, although many can develop in early adulthood.

- Animal Type (example: snakes) and Blood-Injection-Injury Type (example: fear of needles) phobias typically begin in childhood.

- Situational Type (example: being in a closet) phobias, like specific phobias in general, tend to develop in childhood, with a second "peak" in the mid-20s.

Most phobias persist for years or even decades if left untreated.

Fear of animals

Fear of animals is called **zoophobia**. Fear of domestic animals such as cats and dogs is the most common kind of zoophobia. Rats and mice are two of the other most feared animals. Zoophobia can be inconvenient if the phobia involves animals that are popular pets. Most other animals are avoidable simply by not attending zoos, circuses, animal parks, or animal sanctuaries. There are many subtypes of zoophobia. For example, a person with **ornithophobia** has a fear of birds and may be too terrified to go outside for fear of encountering one.

Fear of places

Some people with phobias fear particular places, especially high places or enclosed spaces. A severe fear of heights is called **acrophobia**. Like many other phobias, being afraid of heights is sometimes an appropriate response. Many people are fearful of standing on a mountaintop. However, people with acrophobia fear heights even when they are inside a tall building.

Claustrophobia is a crippling fear of enclosed spaces. Those who suffer from claustrophobia may feel anxious in elevators, cars, closets, airplanes, or even when pulling clothing over their head. Symptoms are similar to those of other phobias and may include excessive sweating or clamminess, rapid breathing and heartbeat, or nausea and dizziness.

Fear of flying is known as **aerophobia** or aviophobia. It is more than concern about airline safety. People with the phobia experience panic attacks that keep them from visiting loved ones or taking vacations. Many who fear flying are afraid of being "closed in" on the plane or unable to escape–symptoms quite similar to those of claustrophobia. A feeling of lack of control often accompanies a fear of flying as well.

A number of people who are afraid to fly experience their fear at different times during a flight. Some are fearful of takeoff; others panic if there is turbulence; still others are afraid of landing or the moment after the plane has landed when everyone stands in the aisles to deplane.

TEENS SPEAK

I Couldn't Get on an Airplane

I won first place at the science fair for my school, and then for the school district. The next step was to bring my project to the state competition. I was psyched. The trouble was, the competition was in the state capitol and I lived about six hours away by car. Part of the award for winning district included airplane tickets for a flight to the competition with one of my parents.

I knew what would happen. Last year we tried to visit my uncle. When I got on the plane, I started sweating and everything seemed kind of blurry. It was as if I were looking at everything through a tunnel. It really seemed as if the cabin was getting smaller and smaller, and I couldn't figure out how all of us would fit if the shrinking continued.

I started having difficulty breathing. Then I started screaming. It was so embarrassing, but I couldn't help it! I needed to get off that plane. I really had to get off the plane. The flight attendant was really, really nice. She came over and asked my mom if we would come with her and she got me off the plane. She offered me a mask that would give me oxygen from a tank. I sat in the airport and tried not to think about that shrinking plane.

A few minutes later, my mom came over and said we were going to take a train instead. She tried to convince me it was okay, but I knew I had ruined the trip for everyone.

So when I won the district competition, I wasn't happy. It was cool to win, and I had worked hard for it. But I knew there was no way I was getting on a plane. I was afraid I'd miss the competition because of it, until my parents made plans to drive me there.

Later, my parents talked to me and said they had found a therapist who could help me. I didn't want to be a freak, but I kept thinking about almost missing the competition. I didn't want to go through that again. I agreed to talk to the guy. It turns out that I have a phobia, a fear of flying. He told me it was common and didn't mean there was something wrong with me. It is a mental disorder that I can't help. He gave me some medication to take before flying, but he thought after all the talking we had done, I probably wouldn't need it!

DO YOU EXPERIENCE PHOBIAS?

For those who suffer from phobias, their fears may be so serious that they cannot do everyday things. They may have a hard time talking to people at school or be unable to visit a friend because of the friend's pet dog. If these worries keep you from doing everyday things, they may be signs of a phobia. You should talk to a doctor about these fears, because phobias are treatable.

DIAGNOSIS AND TREATMENT

People are diagnosed with a phobia only if the fear is unwarranted and impacts their life negatively. Most people who suffer from phobias recognize their fears are out of proportion to the danger, but that knowledge doesn't reduce their fears.

Some mental health professionals are trained specifically to treat phobias. Therapists try to eliminate the phobic part of the fear and replace it with a more appropriate level of concern for safety. They may also prescribe medications that can treat the panic attacks associated with phobias. However, medications do not address the behaviors that cause the phobia.

Traditional therapy for many mental disorders usually involves talking about the problem, developing insights, and recognizing the existence of choices in handling the problem. Traditional therapy doesn't help with phobias, because the fears are irrational. People who have phobias often know how unreasonable their fears are. Only with the aid of some form of therapy that reaches their **subconscious** (the part of the mind below the level of awareness) can these illogical fears be removed.

Types of therapy

Effective treatments for phobias include **hypnotherapy** and **visualization therapy.** Hypnotherapy uses relaxation and positive thoughts to change perceptions of the object of fear. **Hypnosis** is a trancelike state that is brought about by the individual or a trained therapist. The National Board for Certified Clinical Hypnotherapists (NBCCH) defines a **trance** as a state of relaxation in which attention is narrowly focused and relatively free of distractions. Attention may be focused internally (on thoughts) or externally (on the subject of the phobia).

In hypnotherapy, the therapist makes suggestions to encourage thoughts, feelings, and behaviors that may aid a person with a phobia in neutralizing the object of his or her fears. Hypnosis helps to relax people so that they are more open to suggestions. Some feel as if they are literally experiencing what is being suggested. For example, while the individual is in the trancelike state, the therapist might describe an encounter with the object of the phobia. The person with phobia may imagine the encounter almost as if it were really happening—but without fear. When the hypnotic trance ends, many people experience some relief the next time they encounter their phobia.

Visualization therapy is a form of self-hypnosis. It involves developing a mental picture using all of the senses—vision, hearing, smell, touch, and even taste. Another term for this kind of therapy is **creative visualization,** which was the subject of a book of the same name written by Shakti Gawain in 1978. In creative visualization, the person with the phobia imagines what he or she would like to have happen—

perhaps finding enclosed spaces or airplane travel unthreatening. After focusing on the imagined image again and again, it becomes reality.

See also: Anxiety Disorders, Common Types; Related Disorders

FURTHER READING
Gallo, Donald R. *What Are You Afraid Of?: Stories About Phobias.* Somerville, Mass.: Candlewick Press, 2007.

■ POST-TRAUMATIC STRESS DISORDER (PTSD)

An anxiety disorder that affects survivors of such traumatic events as war, terrorist attacks, torture, natural disasters, automobile accidents, airplane crashes, childhood neglect, and violent assaults like rape. Not everyone involved in a traumatic event experiences post-traumatic stress disorder (PTSD). According to the National Institute of Mental Health 7.7 million Americans suffer from PTSD.

SYMPTOMS

PTSD causes physical as well as psychological symptoms. According to a 2004 statement by the National Center for PTSD, physicians often treat these symptoms without being aware that they stem from PTSD. These symptoms most often develop within three months of the traumatic event, though they may not appear for many years. In fact, it takes some people with PTSD months or years—even with professional help—before they realize that their symptoms are related to an event that happened years ago. In any case, the symptoms can be severe enough and last long enough to significantly affect daily life.

Physical symptoms may include

- increased blood pressure
- rapid heart rate or breathing
- muscle tension
- headaches
- gastrointestinal difficulties such as nausea or diarrhea
- immune system problems
- dizziness
- discomfort in other parts of the body

Psychological symptoms may include

- dissociation (losing a sense of reality)
- extreme emotional numbing (inability to feel emotion)
- extreme attempts to avoid disturbing memories (such as through substance use)
- hyper-arousal (panic attacks, rage, extreme irritability)
- severe anxiety (debilitating worry, compulsions, or obsessions)
- severe depression (loss of the ability to feel hope, pleasure, or interest)
- delayed or developmental regression (in children) in such areas as toilet training, motor skills, or language
- intrusive re-experiencing (terrifying memories, nightmares, or flashbacks)

Flashbacks

Many people with PTSD repeatedly re-experience the ordeal in the form of **flashbacks,** memories of previous experiences that are vivid, realistic, and often frightening. Flashbacks can be so dramatic that the sufferer may truly believe he or she is reliving the traumatic time, losing all sense of reality.

Flashbacks are often caused by **triggers.** Triggers are events or objects that remind the sufferer about the trauma they experienced. Anniversaries of the event may also trigger symptoms. Most people with PTSD try to avoid any reminders or thoughts of the ordeal.

Complications

PTSD is complicated by the fact that it frequently occurs at the same time as related disorders such as depression, substance abuse, and memory loss (amnesia). The likelihood of a successful treatment increases when these other conditions are appropriately diagnosed and treated. The disorder is also associated with impairment of the ability to function in social or family life, including occupational instability, marital problems and divorces, family discord, and difficulties in parenting.

RISK FACTORS

The severity of the traumatic event and how long the event lasted appear to be factors in the development of PTSD. According to the

Mayo Clinic, other factors that may increase the likelihood of developing PTSD include

- a previous history of depression or other emotional disorder
- a previous history of physical or sexual abuse
- a family history of anxiety
- early separation from parents
- being part of a dysfunctional family
- alcohol or drug abuse

Young people

Three factors have been shown to increase the likelihood that children will develop PTSD: the severity of the traumatic event, parental reaction to the event, and physical proximity to the event. In general, most studies find that children and adolescents who report the most severe traumas also report the highest levels of PTSD symptoms. Family support and parental coping have also been shown to affect PTSD symptoms in children. According to a 2004 report by the National Center for PTSD, children and adolescents with greater family support and less parental distress have lower levels of PTSD symptoms. Finally, children and adolescents who live far from the place where the traumatic event took place report less distress.

HISTORY AND RATES

PTSD is not a new disorder, even though it was not formally recognized as a psychiatric diagnosis until 1980. According to the National Center for PTSD, written accounts of similar symptoms date back to ancient times, and there is clear documentation of the disorder in medical literature starting with an account of a PTSD-like disorder known as "Da Costa's Syndrome" during the U.S. Civil War. Descriptions of post-traumatic stress symptoms can also be found in the medical literature on combat veterans of World War II and Holocaust survivors.

After the Vietnam War ended in 1975, scientists began thorough research and documentation of PTSD. According to the research, about 30 percent of the men and women who have spent time in war zones experience PTSD. An additional 20 to 25 percent have had partial PTSD at some point in their lives. The National Center for PTSD reported in 2003 that more than half of all male Vietnam veterans and almost half of all female veterans have experienced "clinically serious stress reaction symptoms." PTSD has also been detected among veterans of the Persian Gulf War of 1991. Some studies suggest that as many 20 percent of soldiers returning from the wars in Iraq and Afghanistan suffer from PTSD.

PTSD is not only a problem for veterans, however. It occurs in people of all ages, cultural groups, and socioeconomic levels. The National Institute of Mental Health reported in 2004 that an estimated 7.8 percent of Americans experience PTSD at some point in their lives, with women (10.4 percent) twice as likely as men (5 percent) to develop PTSD. About 3.6 percent of U.S. adults aged 18 to 54 (5.2 million people) have PTSD during the course of a given year. This represents a small portion of those who have experienced at least one traumatic event; 60.7 percent of men and 51.2 percent of women reported at least one traumatic event.

Young people
A few researchers have studied rates of exposure and PTSD in children and adolescents. The National Center for PTSD reported in 2004 that these studies indicate 15 to 43 percent of girls and 14 to 43 percent of boys have experienced at least one traumatic event in their lifetime. Of the children and adolescents who experienced a trauma, 3 to 15 percent of the girls and 1 to 6 percent of the boys could be diagnosed with PTSD.

TREATMENTS AND COPING SKILLS
PTSD treatment usually involves a combination of medications and therapy to control anxiety. There is no cure. However, some treatments, including group therapy and exposure therapy, have proved especially helpful. **Exposure therapy** is a form of therapy in which a survivor confronts feelings or anxieties about a traumatic event by reliving it in a therapy situation. Studies have also shown that medications help ease associated symptoms of depression and anxiety, including sleeplessness. The most widely used drug treatments for PTSD are the **selective serotonin reuptake inhibitors** (SSRI) medications, such as Prozac and Zoloft.

If distress caused by a past traumatic event persistently affects your life, seeing your doctor is a necessary first step. The Mayo Clinic offers the following tips on dealing with PTSD:

■ Follow the doctor's instructions carefully. Although it may take a while to feel the effects of therapy, hang in there. You'll be better off in the long run.

■ Take care of yourself. Get enough rest, eat a balanced diet, exercise, and take time to relax. Avoid caffeine and nicotine, which can worsen anxiety. Don't turn to alcohol or unprescribed drugs for relief.

■ Break the cycle. When you feel anxious, take a brisk walk or delve into a hobby to refocus.

■ Talk to someone. Share your problems with a friend or counselor who can help you gain perspective. Ask your doctor about support groups in your area for people who have post-traumatic stress disorder.

See also: Anxiety Disorders, Common Types

FURTHER READING
Thomas, Peggy. *Post Traumatic Stress Disorder.* Diseases and Disorders. Farmington Hills, Mich.: Lucent Books, 2007.

■ PSYCHOTHERAPIES, KINDS OF
Various methods by which mental health professionals treat those suffering from emotional, behavioral, and mental disorders. It is through psychotherapy that patients learn how their feelings, thoughts, behaviors, and emotions affect their lives and the lives of those around them. Through psychotherapy, individuals learn various coping skills, such as stress management and anger management. Psychotherapy can last months or years, depending on the severity of the mental disorder.

Studies show that different methods of psychotherapy can help those suffering from various mental disorders, especially phobias (irrational fears of specific situations), stress-related maladies, grief, marital problems, and some forms of depression. Patients with more severe problems recover at a much slower rate than those with less severe cases.

THE FIRST STEP
Getting help for an emotional, mental, or behavioral problem might require some research. The hard part is taking the first step to find

help. There are a number of professionals who deal with mental health issues. Some are behavior therapists; others specialize in drug and alcohol treatment. Finding the right treatment for a specific disorder can go a long way in combating the problem. While psychotherapy can be a long, gradual process, over time, patients should begin to feel

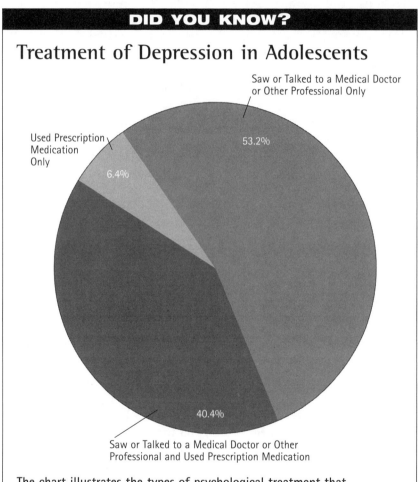

DID YOU KNOW?

Treatment of Depression in Adolescents

Saw or Talked to a Medical Doctor or Other Professional Only

Used Prescription Medication Only

53.2%

6.4%

40.4%

Saw or Talked to a Medical Doctor or Other Professional and Used Prescription Medication

The chart illustrates the types of psychological treatment that adolescents sought for depression in 2007. Most adolescents saw or talked to a medical doctor or other professional. More than 40 percent of adolescents talked to a mental health professional and used medication to treat their mental disorder.

Source: U.S. Department of Health and Human Services, Substance Abuse & Mental Health Services Administration, 2008.

relief from distress. They will be able to develop more self-assuredness and increased emotional comfort in their performance (for example, in school or in work) and in relationships with other people.

Make no mistake about it—therapy can be difficult and uncomfortable at times. Patients will often experience varying degrees of discomfort as psychotherapy plumbs the root cause of hurt feelings and deep-seated problems. However, with time, psychotherapy can help a person effectively cope with those feelings.

How do you find a therapist? You can either find one on your own, or get a **referral** from a doctor, a health insurance company, a friend, or a family member. Also, many communities have mental health agencies to aid your search. They will be able to provide you with good information on the type of therapy you may need.

Psychotherapy is not cheap, but do not let that stop you or your loved ones from seeking help. Many health insurance plans will help pay to treat members suffering from mental disorders. Also, many clinics, mental health agencies, and mental health professionals often offer sliding-fee scales based on a person's income, according to which those with a lower income pay less than those with a higher income. Occasionally, treatment is free.

Q & A

Question: What can I expect once I begin treatment?

Answer: When you first see a therapist, you likely will visit his or her office. Sessions also can be held in a hospital if one is admitted for treatment. Either way, you will talk with your therapist for 45 to 60 minutes, usually once a week, during each session. During the first meeting the therapist typically asks questions and gathers information about the problem. It might take a few weeks before a therapist evaluates your situation. He or she will then help you work through your problems using various techniques.

PSYCHOSOCIAL AND INDIVIDUAL PSYCHOTHERAPY
Figuring out what type of mental health treatment you need is essential. Some psychotherapy includes social or vocational training. Such *psychosocial* treatments provide support, education, and guidance to patients and their families. A licensed **psychiatrist**, social worker, or

counselor helps treat people who undergo psychosocial treatments. Sometimes two or more professionals will work together.

Often, patients settle on one-on-one psychotherapy with a mental health professional such as a psychiatrist, psychologist, psychiatric social worker, or others. The goal of such **individual psychotherapy** is to help patients understand their behavior while learning how to control or correct such behavior. Those suffering from a variety of mental disorders, such as phobias, **bipolar disorder,** depression, or **eating disorders,** often find relief in individual psychotherapy.

MENTAL HEALTH TREATMENTS

There are many kinds of psychological techniques used to treat a person suffering from emotional or behavioral problems. Some of these, noted here in alphabetical order only, include the following:

- **art therapy:** Art therapy uses a person's creative abilities to help express feelings, emotions, and thoughts through drawing, writing, sculpting, painting, or music.

- **behavior therapy:** This type of therapy changes a person's unhealthy behavior by using a system of rewards. Behavior therapy also desensitizes patients, allowing them to change the way they live their lives.

- **cognitive therapy:** Cognitive therapy seeks to correct a person's thinking (cognitive) patterns that could lead to unhealthy feelings and behavior. The goal is to recognize negative thoughts and replace them with more appropriate thought patterns and behaviors.

- **cognitive behavior therapy (CBT):** To combat depression, this combination of cognitive and behavior therapies helps a person not only understand and identify negative views and unhealthy behavior but also to replace those thoughts and behaviors with healthy and positive ones.

- **dialectical behavior therapy:** This type of therapy teaches a patient such skills as **stress** management and anger management. These coping skills regulate a person's emotions and help improve relationships with others.

■ **drug therapy:** Using prescribed medication helps some people with emotional and mental disorders.

■ **electroconvulsive treatment (ECT):** Doctors will prescribe ECT to treat major, treatment-resistant cases of depression, especially those cases that do not respond

DID YOU KNOW?

Treatment of Depression in Adults

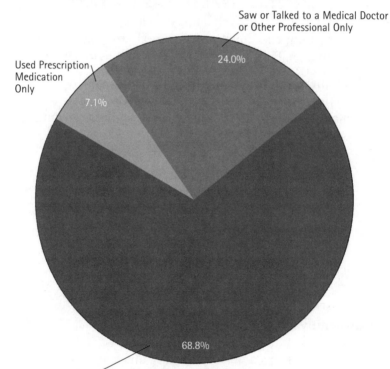

Saw or Talked to a Medical Doctor or Other Professional Only

24.0%

Used Prescription Medication Only

7.1%

68.8%

Saw or Talked to a Medical Doctor or Other Professional and Used Prescription Medication

The chart illustrates the types of psychological treatment that adults sought for depression in 2007. Most saw or talked to a medical doctor or other professional. The majority of adults also used prescription medications to treat their mental disorder.

Source: U.S. Department of Health and Human Services, Substance Abuse & Mental Health Services Administration, 2008.

to medications, or where there are life-threatening suicidal behaviors, **delusions,** or **hallucinations.**

■ **exposure therapy:** Therapists will deliberately expose patients to something that upsets them in an attempt to teach them how to cope with similar stressors.

■ **family therapy:** This type of therapy helps families understand the problems that someone in the family might have. The goal is to improve the way in which family members interact with one another.

■ **group therapy:** In this treatment, qualified mental health professionals bring together groups of people who share the same disorder or problem to discuss coping with or resolving their problems.

■ **interpersonal therapy:** Individuals who go through interpersonal therapy want to overcome depression and improve their interpersonal skills and relationships with family, friends, and colleagues.

■ **marriage counseling:** Also known as couples therapy, marriage counseling seeks to give couples—married and not—the opportunity to work through problems by talking and other techniques.

■ **play therapy:** Generally reserved for young children with varying developmental levels, play therapy allows children experiencing problems to more easily express their emotions and feelings.

■ **psychoanalysis:** This in-depth therapy helps patients dig deep into past memories and events to understand their current feelings and behavior.

■ **psychodynamic psychotherapy:** This type of therapy focuses on increasing a patient's awareness of unconscious thoughts and behaviors. Psychodynamic psychotherapy offers a patient the ability to assess his or her motivations and resolve conflicts.

■ **psychoeducation:** This therapy involves teaching people and family members about a mental disorder and how to treat it. Through psychoeducation, patients learn coping skills and problem-solving strategies to reduce discomfort, distress, anxiety, and confusion.

Q & A

Question: Are there are any risks associated with psychotherapy?

Answer: Although there is little risk in going through psychotherapy, the process can be uncomfortable. It can bring to the forefront certain feelings, memories, and emotions that you may have wanted to avoid. Still, the coping mechanisms you learn through the psychotherapy certainly can benefit you in the long run.

See also: Treatment of Anxiety Disorders; Treatment of Mood Disorders

FURTHER READING

Backman, Margaret E. *Coping With Choosing a Therapist: A Young Person's Guide to Counseling and Psychotherapy.* New York: Rosen Publishing, 1993.

Stallard, Paul, *Think Good—Feel Good: A Cognitive Behaviour Therapy Workbook for Children.* West Sussex, U.K.: Wiley, 2002.

■ RELATED DISORDERS

Specific mental disorders or conditions related to or accompanying the primary disorder. Mental health professionals classify **psychiatric** conditions into different groups. They often diagnose patients with anxiety disorders, dissociative disorders, substance abuse disorders, **eating disorders,** and personality disorders, among others. In each group, however, are related disorders, most of which have their own symptoms and causes.

For example, under the general diagnosis of anxiety disorder, a patient might suffer related disorders such as panic attacks, social phobias, or obsessive-compulsive behavior. The symptoms for each related disorder are different, but the general disorder is the same.

Q & A

Question: What does it mean if someone is afraid to go out?

Answer: This is called **agoraphobia,** a specific type of anxiety disorder. It involves an intense fear of any open or public place where escape is difficult. People who suffer from agoraphobia generally do not leave their homes or travel in a car, bus, or airplane. There are approximately 1.8 million American adults who suffer from this related disorder.

Other examples are **anorexia nervosa** and **bulimia nervosa**, which are different types of eating disorders. Depression and bipolar disorder are two types of mood disorders. Below is a list of several types of mental conditions and their related disorders:

Anxiety Disorders

- acute stress disorder
- panic disorder
- agoraphobia without history of panic disorder
- social phobia
- specific phobia
- obsessive-compulsive disorder
- post-traumatic stress disorder (PTSD)
- generalized anxiety disorder (GAD)

Childhood Disorders

- attention-deficit/hyperactivity disorder
- Asperger's syndrome
- autistic disorder
- conduct disorder
- oppositional defiant disorder
- separation anxiety disorder
- Tourette's syndrome

Eating Disorders

- anorexia nervosa
- bulimia nervosa
- binge eating disorder

Mood Disorders

- major depressive disorder
- bipolar disorder (manic-depressive disorder)

- cyclothymic disorder
- dysthymic disorder
- seasonal affective disorder (SAD)

Cognitive Disorders

- delirium
- multi-infarct dementia
- dementia associated with alcoholism
- dementia of the Alzheimer type
- dementia

DID YOU KNOW?

Drug Use Among Persons 12 Years Old and Older

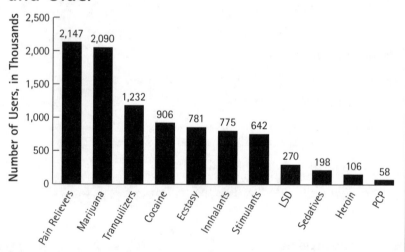

Substance abuse is a major problem with which many individuals must grapple. The abuse of one type of drug may lead to the use or abuse of a related substance, such as marijuana use, alcohol use, and the use of inhalants or stimulants. The graph above charts the number of individuals 12 years old and older who abused drugs (illegal and prescription) in 2007.

Source: Substance Abuse and Mental Health Services Administration (SAMHSA), 2007.

TEENS SPEAK

My Mom's a Hoarder

My name is Jessica and you will never come to my house. It's not because I don't like you; it's because I'm embarrassed. What's the problem? My mother is a "pack rat," a person who keeps anything and everything. She said she "collects" things. I know better. She has stacked old newspapers, some dating back to 1990, up to the ceiling. I haven't seen the kitchen table in years. It's crammed with food, boxes, books, old cell phones, ancient bank statements, and all sorts of other junk.

The living room is a mess. Magazines, tables, chairs, boxes, and bags clutter the room. It is tough to find a place to sit. My mother's room is a disaster area. Piles of clothes, stacks of books, shoes, and other debris clutter the floor. Let's not even talk about the garage. I haven't been able to walk from one end of the garage to the other in more than five years. The only two rooms in the house that are neat are the upstairs bathroom and my room—and that's because I keep them tidy.

It wasn't always like this. When I was a young child, maybe five or six years old, I remember that our house was clean and neat. The backyard was perfectly landscaped. Relatives and family friends used to come over all the time. My aunt and uncle came over every Saturday night and played cards with mom and dad while I was upstairs in the bedroom. About 10 years ago, things started to change. My dad walked out.

My mom didn't start "collecting" things all at once. It was gradual. She'd bring something home from a tag sale or the store and put it on the floor. She'd never unwrap the item or use it. It just sat and took up space. She'd buy baby clothes even though there wasn't a baby in the house. "Oh, someone will need it. Someone's always having a baby," she would say. Well, the clothes are still here.

The dining room was the first place to become cluttered. After dad left, we didn't really use the dining room all that much. We'd eat our meals in the living room in front of the television. Apparently, Mom thought that since we were no longer using the dining room, it was okay to put stuff in there. Soon, it became a dumping ground. Soon, other rooms suffered the same fate.

At first, I didn't think anything was wrong. But when I got a little older and started visiting the homes of friends, I knew that what was happening in my home was not normal. By the time I was 12, my mother's "collecting" was out of control. Mom gets angry any time I suggest that we clean the house. "Mom," I would say, "Why do you need shopping lists from years ago? Why do you hang on to clothing that doesn't fit anymore? Can't we return all these soda cans to the store?" Each time I questioned Mom, or suggested that we clean the house, she would get defensive.

I soon learned that my mom was a hoarder. I was informed that hoarding is an obsessive-compulsive disorder (OCD), which I know now is an anxiety disorder.

We all get anxious from time to time. Sometimes though, anxiety can get out of control, and that's what happened to my mom.

Hoarding is one type of OCD. People who suffer from compulsive hoarding, like my mom, often don't see it as a problem. Hoarders collect items because they think those items have some value, or they might use them at some point. A person might hoard items because they represent happier times or remind them of a loved one. Like my mom, people who hoard may feel safe when they are surrounded by the things they collect.

I finally convinced my mother that she had to seek treatment. I told her that collecting so much junk was unhealthy and dangerous. I'm going off to college next year. I can't wait. I can't wait to have friends over to my dorm room. I can't wait to leave all this junk behind.

Treatment seems to be helping. Little by little, my mom is throwing away the junk she doesn't need. The psychologist says it might take years for Mom to get over her compulsion. I just hope that she does.

SOMATOFORM DISORDERS

Somatoform disorders are any psychological conditions in which a person feels physical pain even though that pain and its symptoms do not actually exist. At first these symptoms tend to be related to a specific physical ailment, but medical test results eventually reveal that the person's physical health is normal. Somatoform patients are often worried about their physical health because their symptoms are similar to other known illnesses and may last for several years. Most people tend to think that those who suffer from this disorder are fakers or **hypochondriacs**; however, the pain they feel is real to them.

Related disorders include somatization disorder, which is characterized by somatic symptoms that cannot be adequately explained; conversion disorder, which is characterized by a sudden loss of neurological function, such as becoming mute; pain disorder; hypochondria; and body dysmorphic disorder, characterized by a focus on a physical defect that is not evident to others.

ADJUSTMENT DISORDER

Whenever a person changes a job, gets married, or goes to a new school, there is a period where he or she must adjust to a new environment or different life. Most people adjust to such situations within a few months. Many, however, do not. They suffer from an adjustment disorder.

Adjustment disorder is related to anxiety disorder, specifically those made worse by stress. Some people might become anxious, depressed, and even suicidal. People suffer from adjustment disorder because they no longer go through their daily routines, such as going to the same school or seeing their old friends.

Most adults get better within just a few months. Teenagers, however, might need more time. Treatment can lessen the impact of an adjustment disorder, preventing it from becoming a serious problem. How do you know if you have an adjustment disorder? Some symptoms include: a change in some routine accompanied by sadness, hopelessness, nervousness, anxiety, and trouble sleeping.

GRIEVING

Grieving—the intense sorrow that someone feels for the loss of a loved one—is a fact of life, and all of us go through the process at one point or another. When someone you are close to dies, there is always something that reminds you of them. Sometimes the pain of such a loss can last for months or even years.

People also may grieve over things other than death. They may feel grief over giving a baby up for adoption, for example, or over the loss of a pet. Just when you think you have gotten over the loss of someone you loved, an anniversary, birthday, or holiday may bring back memories of that person. Although experiencing such sad feelings are normal, these emotional reactions can last for days and even weeks at a time. You might feel sad, lonely, or angry. You might have nightmares, crying spells, or trouble eating.

Although many 20th-century experts, such as Elizabeth Kubler-Ross, John Bowlby, and George Engel, identified both specific stages and types of grief, many modern psychologists recommend that a grieving person must

■ accept the reality of the loss, which takes time;

■ work through the pain of the grief, which can be both physical and emotional;

■ adjust to a changed environment, which means accepting the world as it is.

See also: Anxiety Disorders, Symptoms of; Bipolar Disorder; Depression and Mood Disorder, Causes of; Depression and Substance Abuse; Phobias

FURTHER READING
Ghaemi, Nassir S. *Mood Disorders: A Practical Guide.* 2nd ed. Philadelphia: Lippincott Williams & Wilkins, 2008.

■ RESILIENCY

The ability to recover from life's setbacks. Everyone experiences difficult times in life. When it comes to mental disorders, resiliency greatly enhances the process of rehabilitation, or treatment.

CHARACTERISTIC AMONG TEENS

Most teenagers "bounce back" from anxiety disorder and depression if they are treated for the disorders. This is true for other sufferers as well, but teens are especially skillful at the personal growth and reflection necessary for recovery. The teen years are a time of great physical and emotional changes. **Introspection,** examining one's emotions and motivations, is common in young people. Because successful treatment for depression generally includes some form of talk therapy, this skill is particularly useful. According to a report released by the National Institute of Mental Health (2000), teens have a high rate of recovery from a single episode of depression. However, one episode of depression puts them at increased risk of future depression.

People are more likely to be resilient if they feel positive about themselves and valued by friends and family, have a good perception of themselves (self-esteem), and have the support of friends or family. A resilient person is likely to have good social skills, intelligence, and independence.

Some people believe that external forces, such as the actions of other people or situations over which one has no control, determine how life turns out. Others recognize that their personal choices and attitudes can make a difference. This sense of personal control is essential to a successful recovery.

Having the characteristics of a resilient person doesn't guarantee that one will recover quickly from stressful situations, just as the absence of these qualities doesn't mean he or she won't recover quickly. People need to experience some success in recovering from depression before they realize they can be successful.

Fact Or Fiction?

Talking about depression only makes it worse.

The Facts: Talking with friends who are depressed can help them recognize that they may need professional help. If you offer friendship, concern, and support without judgment, you can encourage your friends to seek the treatment they need. Remember that even though you can help, your friends will also need to talk with a professional to begin the recovery process.

STRATEGIES FOR BOUNCING BACK

For those suffering from anxiety or depression, it is important to get professional help from a therapist they trust. A doctor may also prescribe medications. If medications are prescribed, it is important to take them as directed to begin the process of treating the depression.

Depression and anxiety disorders are mental disorders that require professional treatment. However, the same things people do to avoid mental disorders can be part of a strategy for bouncing back from an anxiety disorder or depression. Suggestions for avoiding or healing depression or anxiety disorders include the following:

- Seek out the activities that make you feel better.
- Avoid spending too much time alone.
- Talk to your family and friends.
- Get help with your workload when you need it.

It can also help to:

- Eat healthy foods.
- Stay away from alcohol or drugs.
- Exercise at least three times a week.
- Get enough rest (sleep at regular hours).
- Find time to relax every day.
- When you are feeling stress, try to breathe deeply.
- Think often about the good things in your life.
- Trust that things will work for your good.
- Learn new and better ways to take care of problems.

One important element in recovering from depression or anxiety is building and maintaining a social support network. Those who suffer from depression or anxiety may have difficulty talking with people about how they feel. If they are around positive and supportive people, they find it easier and more productive to express themselves. It is difficult to get better if one is surrounded by people who are pessimistic or abusing drugs or alcohol. It may also be difficult if family and friends dismiss one's feelings or have a negative perspective.

Support groups can help people with a mental disorder realize they are not alone. Many people acquire strategies for dealing with their disorder by talking with those who are struggling with similar issues. Discussing which strategies work and which do not can be helpful. You can find a support group by looking in the phone book, searching the Web, or asking a therapist or guidance counselor for suggestions.

The Internet, books, and CDs can also promote resiliency. Some audiobooks help listeners build self-confidence, overcome negative thinking, or learn relaxation techniques. These techniques may be helpful in recovery. Searching the Web using terms like "depression help" or "anxiety healing" will bring up links to dozens of Web sites. Some may be helpful, while others may not. The act of searching for help, however, can be a positive step in recovering. You will also find a list of resources at the end of this book.

If you are suffering from depression or anxiety, know that you are not alone. It is easy to feel you are the only person who feels the way you do, when the reality is there are thousands—even millions—of people who are experiencing similar troubles. A professional therapist will be able to tell you why you are not alone and that recovery is possible. Such positive truths are important to recognize, although depression or anxiety may make them difficult to accept.

TEENS SPEAK

Getting Better Every Day

The first sign something wasn't right was when my coach asked me to take a break from the team. I had been a starter for our school football team since I was a sophomore. Coach took me aside and said he thought I should talk with a counselor about what was going on in my life.

DID YOU KNOW?

Fish May Prevent Pregnancy Blues

Omega-3 essential fatty acid, a beneficial oil found in certain kinds of seafood, may significantly reduce the risk of depression during pregnancy.

Source: American Psychiatry Association, 2009.

I had missed practices because I slept through them. I wasn't making good plays because I couldn't keep any of them straight in my head. When my teammates tried to talk to me, I yelled at them or didn't say anything at all. Inside I was constantly worried, always thinking about what bad thing could happen next. I didn't realize I was experiencing general anxiety disorder.

I talked to our school counselor about my worries. He helped me come up with a plan to help myself feel better. He told me that I was resilient, that I could bounce back from feeling as bad as I did. Together, we looked at the choices I was making in my life. He pointed out I was drinking a lot of caffeine and that was adding to my nervousness. The caffeine also made it hard for me to fall asleep at night so I was overtired. I was also eating a lot of foods made with refined sugar—junk food—like potato chips, donuts, and cupcakes. My counselor told me those foods could affect my emotions, making me feel really energetic for a while and then extremely tired and even sad when the effects wore off. We agreed I would make changes in my diet. I would start bringing a healthy lunch from home. I would drink more water and, at the very least, non-caffeinated beverages.

My counselor also told me that exercise could help me feel calm. Since I was an athlete already, we agreed I would simply go for a walk around the neighborhood on days I didn't have practice or a game.

After talking with my counselor, I was able to see how much better I felt just telling someone about my fears. I think I kept my worries and fears inside me, trying to seem strong. Instead of seeming strong, I ended up an irritable mess. I decided I would hang out with my best friend more often, even just to do homework. Spending time with friends and letting them know how I really feel was part of my plan to feel better.

My counselor also told me if making these changes in my life didn't help much, it was possible I would need to take some medication. The medication would help my brain chemistry work better so I wouldn't be worried and scared all the time.

I was lucky. Once I stopped drinking so much caffeine and eating so much sugar and started talking to my friends and teammates about my fears, I felt courageous and strong. I went walking almost every day. Sometimes I'd listen to music, sometimes I'd just walk and think. I was able to sleep better. All these changes, combined with the work I did with my counselor, made me feel calm and peaceful most of the time. I didn't need to take medication. It's not that I stopped worrying, it's that I now worry much less and usually only about things that most people worry about (like tests or big games). It turns out I am resilient, and I like it!

Having a resilient personality may make it easier to feel better once professional treatment has begun. Those who recover easily from life's setbacks may already have some of the skills necessary for recovery. Taking care of oneself physically and emotionally is one of the most important things a person can do to avoid or heal from depression or anxiety disorders.

See also: Risk Factors for Depression

FURTHER READING

Bellenir, Karen. *Mental Health Information for Teens: Health Tips About Mental Health and Mental Illness.* 1st ed. Detroit: Omnigraphics, 2001.

Damon, William, and Nancy Eisenberg. *Social, Emotional, and Personality Development.* Vol. 3, *Handbook of Child Psychology,* 5th ed. Hoboken, N.J.: Wiley, 2000.

Shapiro, Lawrence E., and Robin K. Sprague. *The Relaxation & Stress Reduction Workbook for Kids: Help for Children to Cope With Stress, Anxiety & Transitions.* Oakland, Calif.: New Harbinger Publications, 2009.

■ RISK FACTORS FOR DEPRESSION

Circumstances that increase a person's chances of developing a mental disorder caused by a chemical imbalance in the brain, the most common symptoms or signs of which are long-lasting feelings of hopelessness and despair, lack of energy, and, sometimes, suicidal tendencies. Mental health professionals have isolated a number of risk factors for depression, which exist before the disorder develops, although not everyone with these risk factors for depression becomes depressed.

A vulnerability to depression appears to run in some families. Also, research suggests that people who experience a traumatic event or life change have a greater risk for depression. An illness, such as stroke or heart attack, or medication prescribed for certain illnesses may also place a person at risk for depression.

A symptom is a sign that something is wrong; it is a result of a disorder. Some risk factors may also be symptoms of depression. For example, substance abuse increases the likelihood of depression. Substance abuse is also a common symptom of depression. Depression is a physiological illness, but environmental factors and lifestyle choices can affect how one's body responds to stress. While controlling the chemical imbalances that most mental health professionals associate with depression, people can also make choices that help prevent or ease depression.

TOBACCO USE AND ADOLESCENTS

Tobacco use usually begins in adolescence. Moreover, tobacco use seems to be a gateway to other substance addictions and to some mental disorders. In 2007, researchers at Columbia University concluded that smoking cigarettes might make teens more prone to depression, alcohol abuse, and illegal drug use.

In their report, *Tobacco: The Smoking Gun,* researchers at Columbia University's National Center on Addiction and Substance Abuse, say that teens who smoke are nine times more likely to abuse alcohol and 13 times more likely to abuse illegal drugs than teens who do not smoke.

Every day, an estimated 4,000 teens in the United States take a drag on a cigarette for the first time. The report states that twice as many teen smokers suffer symptoms of depression compared to teens who do not smoke. Moreover, other studies link smoking at a young age to panic attacks and general anxiety disorders.

In addition, teen smokers between the ages of 12 and 17 are five times more likely to drink alcohol. Teen smokers are nine times more likely to fit the clinical definition of a person who abuses alcohol compared to teens who do not smoke.

Teen smokers are also 13 times more likely to smoke marijuana than nonsmoking teens. The report also states that children who start smoking before they turn 13 are three times as likely to engage in **binge drinking** as are nonsmokers. They are also 15 times as likely to smoke marijuana and seven times more likely to abuse other illegal drugs compared to children who do not smoke.

People with depression may use drugs or alcohol because they think it might help them feel better. Or they may abuse drugs or alcohol to hurt themselves. Because depression and substance abuse so often occur at the same time, mental health professionals consider substance abuse a risk factor for depression. Substance abuse is an example of a behavior that may be both a risk factor *and* a symptom of depression.

Substance abuse can also increase the likelihood of suicide. According to the NAMI (2003), teenagers who abuse drugs or alcohol are more likely to progress from suicidal thoughts to suicide attempts. If depression is added to the equation, substance abuse becomes even more deadly.

Q & A

Question: I'm shy and I have had a hard time making friends. I feel really bad about myself and I'm lonely. How can I make friends with the kids at my new school?

Answer: The most important thing you can do is enjoy your own company. If you like yourself, other people will be more likely to realize you are likeable. That said, there are some steps you can take to make new friends. Spending time with people with similar interests is always a good way to make friends. If you enjoy playing a musical instrument or doing crafts, you may want to join an after-school band or an art club. Keep in mind that many people are nervous about making friends, so you are not alone.

ISOLATION

Being alone can be a symptom of depression or it can be a risk factor contributing to its development. Those suffering from depression may find it easy to talk themselves into believing they are not worthy of being in the company of others. They may believe they will only drag their friends down. They are also likely to imagine that no one wants to be with them, because they are depressed. In addition, they may lack the energy or desire to spend time with people. Those who spend too much time alone may begin to believe that they have no friends, no one cares, and they are unlovable. Such thinking can make depression more severe.

Social support is important in recovering from depression. Having the support of family and friends may help reduce the chances of depression. If you are suffering from depression, ask for help from family members or friends. Remember that depression is an illness, not a personal weakness or defect in character. People who care about you will want you to get help to feel better.

TEENS SPEAK

No One Had Any Idea How Lonely I Was

My friends were the popular ones. My best friend was captain of cheerleading and our other friend was class president. We went to the best parties and none of us ever got into trouble. The boys in our group were the hottest, and we were the prettiest. Everything looked great—from the outside.

What no one knew was that when I went home from school, I would stop at the convenience store on the corner and buy a ton of junk food. I would get home, turn on the television to some stupid after–school show, and I would eat and eat and eat.

Sure, I'd chat with my friends online, or talk to them on the phone. Boys called me, too. When anyone wanted to talk to me, I snapped out of it long enough to seem happy. But I felt dead inside. I would sleep, watch television, and eat. Then I started throwing up the food because I didn't want to get fat. We didn't have fat friends. I knew that wasn't an option.

One day my cheerleader friend, Kirsten, wanted to come over. I didn't want to bring her into my house. I didn't want her to see how I was living. I must've been a real mess, because we were sitting in her car in front of my house and I just started crying. It seemed like I couldn't stop talking, I couldn't stop telling her how bad I'd been feeling for so long.

Even though we'd never talked like that before, I was lucky. Her mom was a therapist, so Kirsten called her, and I went over to her house to talk to her mom. Her mom set me up with a therapist she knew who treated teenagers with depression.

It took a couple months for things to get better, but they did. The thing that was really great, besides feeling so much better, was that I think I started being a better person. I was nicer to people who weren't in our crowd, and to those who were. I realized that just because people seem happy on the outside—maybe it seems like they have everything going for them—they could be hurting inside.

INFLUENCE OF PEERS

Adolescence is a time when the influence of friends becomes very important. It is also a time when teens may begin to make their own lifestyle choices instead of following their parents' ideas. Having friends who get into trouble or who are antisocial may increase one's likelihood of developing emotional or behavioral problems. The choices one's friends make may add to one's own risk factors. For example, if one's friends use drugs and alcohol, he or she may feel pressure to do the same, thus increasing the likelihood of depression.

Sometimes a group of friends fall into a pattern of negative thinking that can become quite extreme. It becomes "uncool" to be positive and happy. It is not a sign of weakness to be influenced by those people around you. It is normal, which is why spending time with positive, motivated, and honest people can decrease the chances of experiencing depression.

People can also be at risk for depression because of social isolation. If someone has been the target of teasing or cruelty, he or she may become more easily depressed than others who have not been a target. Any kind of harassment can have a negative effect on mental health. These findings are supported by studies that show the impact of perceived discrimination on children of Asian, Latin American, and Caribbean immigrants. Two additional studies found that perceived discrimination was closely related to symptoms of depression among adults of Mexican origin and Asians.

A report issued by the Surgeon General (1999) focused on the effects of racism on the mental health of African Americans. Its findings indicated that racism and discrimination are stressful events that can place minorities at risk for mental disorders such as depression and anxiety.

TRAUMA AND STRESS

Everyone reacts differently to the stresses of life. What causes one person to lose sleep or become immobilized with hopelessness may be inconsequential to another person. Sometimes, for a very sensitive person, the usual stresses of daily life can be enough to increase the chances of developing depression. Exams at school, tryouts for a play or sports team, or even simple social interactions may be enough to trigger depression in some individuals. Most people, however, are unlikely to experience depression from everyday stresses, although they may get a case of the blues (feeling dejected or gloomy) for a short period of time.

A more likely risk factor for depression is **post-traumatic stress disorder,** or PTSD. PTSD is an anxiety disorder that has strong connections to depression. The National Center for PTSD defines PTSD as a disorder that can occur following the experience or witnessing of life-threatening events such as military combat, natural disasters, terrorist incidents, serious accidents, or violent personal assaults like rape. Specific traumatic events in childhood, especially those that disrupt the family, such as child abuse, can also have serious emotional effects later in life.

One of the most common symptoms of PTSD is depression. The traumatic event as well as other stresses in life can result in a **predisposition,** a tendency or inclination, to developing depression. Once a predisposition has been established, environmental situations such as trauma may cause depression. If someone experiences a horrific event as a young child or even in the more recent past, he or she may be more likely to develop depression.

GENETIC HISTORY

A **genetic** disorder is an illness that is inherited. Like hair or eye color, some physical and mental illnesses are thought to have a genetic, or **hereditary,** component. According to the National Institute for Mental Health (NIMH), early research suggested a strong hereditary component to mental illness. Statistics published by the NIMH in 2003 showed that close relatives of people with depression are more likely to develop depression than those who don't have family members who are depressed. In fact, Drs. Avshalom Caspi and Terrie Moffitt of the University of Wisconsin reported in *Science* (2003) that one particular gene, the "short," or stress-sensitive version, of the **serotonin** transporter gene, doubles the risk of depression following life stresses in early adulthood. After further research, however, scientists at the National Institute of Mental Health today report that the gene might not play a role in depression at all. Scientists now believe that mental disorders such as depression are caused by genetic risk factors in combination with environmental triggers.

Researchers have found no evidence that depression is hereditary. However, they have established that the presence of depression in a family is a risk factor for developing depression. The NIMH explains that although there is strong evidence that mental illness runs in families, no specific gene has been identified for any of the common forms of mental disorders, including depression. Many researchers believe this is due, in part, to the effect of the environment on genes. They recognize that one's genes do not necessarily determine his or her fate. The choices one makes, where he or she lives, and other external forces make a difference in what role genes play.

Fact Or Fiction?

My mother, grandfather, and sister all suffer from depression, so I am going to get it too.

The Facts: If depression seems to run in your family, you may be at greater risk of experiencing it. However, it is also possible that you may never develop depression. Your environment—friends, family, school, work—plays a large part in your chances of developing the disorder. So, even though depression may exist in your family, you may never experience it, if your environment is healthy and supportive.

FAMILY FACTORS AND SOCIAL ENVIRONMENT

In addition to genetics, trauma, and stress, a person's social environment affects the likelihood that he or she will develop depression. How people behave, their relationships, their education, their work, the communities they live in, and how they feel about themselves are also elements of the social environment.

Difficult family events, including divorce or the death of a loved one, can contribute to depression. So can the stresses of living with someone who is struggling with depression, anxiety, or substance abuse. Relationship issues, such as codependency, are more likely to happen where one or more family members is ill. Codependency is a set of compulsive behaviors that family members learn to help them survive in an emotionally painful and stressful environment. Similar stresses may result from friends or people at work who are experiencing anxiety, depression, or related disorders like substance abuse.

COPING WITH RISK FACTORS

The more risk factors a person has, the more likely he or she is to experience depression. However, having one or even several risk factors does not mean that a person will develop depression. In fact, there are many things people can do to decrease the likelihood of depression. They can avoid drugs and alcohol, surround themselves with positive people, get professional help if family members are suffering from depression or other disorders, and take care of themselves mentally and physically. If you or someone you know is experiencing symptoms of depression, remember that it is a treatable disease and help is available.

See also: Anxiety Disorders, Common Types of; Codependency; Depression, Causes of; Genetics of Mood Disorders and Anxiety

FURTHER READING

Kramlinger, Keith, ed. *Mayo Clinic on Depression: Answers to Help You Understand, Recognize and Manage Depression.* Rochester, Minn.: Mayo Clinic, 2002.

Task Force on DSM-IV. *Diagnostic and Statistical Manual of Mental Disorders DSM-IV-TR (Text Revision).* Arlington, Va.: American Psychiatric Publishing, 2000.

■ SEASONAL AFFECTIVE DISORDER (SAD)

A mood disorder characterized by a depression thought to be triggered by a decrease in exposure to sunlight.

Everyone feels down or sluggish sometimes. Some people may even get the "winter blues" when it is too chilly to go outside, so they may feel restless and bored. However, some people experience a more serious mood change when the cold weather rolls around. They may feel like they can't get out of bed in the morning, have no energy, and increased cravings for sweets. They may also feel depressed, showing no interest in everyday activities or in talking to friends. Sometimes, these symptoms are quite severe. This condition is known as seasonal affective disorder, or SAD.

Symptoms of SAD have been documented since the 1800s, but the disorder was not named until the 1980s. Norman Rosenthal, then a researcher at the National Institute for Mental Health (NIMH), gave the disorder its name. SAD is "seasonal" because the mood change occurs during a certain season, and it is "affective," or emotional, because it causes emotional changes in a person.

If SAD is left untreated, people with the disorder may not be able to carry out their day-to-day routines. For others, it is a milder condition, causing a discomfort known as sub-syndromal SAD or winter blues. SAD is often misdiagnosed as hypothyroidism (a disorder of the thyroid gland), hypoglycemia (a disorder involving blood sugar levels), infectious mononucleosis, or other viral infections.

SYMPTOMS

Those who have experienced the following symptoms each winter for at least two years, but always feel better in the spring and summer months, may have SAD. The symptoms are

- depression
- loss of energy
- anxiety
- irritability
- headaches
- increased sleep
- loss of interest in pleasurable things
- overeating, especially foods high in carbohydrates
- weight gain
- difficulty concentrating and processing information

RATES

SAD affects millions of people every winter between September and April, in particular during December, January, and February. According to the U.S. Department of Health and Human Services (DHHS), a less common version of SAD can occur in the summer, but SAD almost always occurs during the winter months in colder climates. In fact, people who live in New Hampshire are about seven times more likely to suffer from SAD than those who live in Florida.

A 2004 report issued by the Cleveland Clinic estimates that 10 to 20 percent of adults in the United States may suffer from a milder form of winter blues. Females over the age of 20 are more likely to suffer from full-blown SAD than males, though SAD can occur in both genders and every age group (older adults are least likely to experience SAD).

CAUSES

Doctors don't know the causes of SAD, but heredity, stress, and the availability of sunlight all play a role. Many people with SAD report at least one close relative with a psychiatric condition, most frequently a severe depressive disorder (55 percent) or alcohol abuse (34 percent), according to NIMH in 2004.

The shorter days and scarce daylight of the winter months are the most common elements thought to cause SAD. The lack of sunlight increases a sleep-related hormone called melatonin. This hormone, which may cause symptoms of depression, is produced at higher levels when it is dark. Therefore, when the days are shorter and darker the production of this hormone increases.

Researchers also suspect that reduced sunlight may disrupt **circadian rhythms,** which regulate the body's internal clock. The circadian rhythms let you know when it is time to sleep and when it is time to wake up. A disruption in the sleep cycle may cause depression.

TREATMENT

Although there's no cure for SAD, there are treatments that successfully manage the condition so that sufferers experience each season in relative safety.

Bright light therapy, or **phototherapy,** has been shown to suppress the brain's secretion of melatonin and reverse the winter depressive symptoms of SAD. Ordinary light bulbs and fittings are not strong enough. The special lights should be at least 10 times the intensity of ordinary domestic lighting. Usual treatment includes exposure from 30 minutes to several hours per day.

Although there have been no research findings to definitively link this therapy with an antidepressant effect, studies do show that many people respond to the treatment. In a 2004 study by the National Alliance for the Mentally Ill, 80 percent of 112 patients improved significantly with light therapy. Antidepressants such as Zoloft and Prozac may also be helpful in treating SAD.

The special lighting device most often used today is a bank of full-spectrum fluorescent lights on a metal reflector and shield with a plastic screen. The intensity of light from this special source is equivalent to the amount of light exposure a person would receive by standing near a window on a sunny spring day. For mild symptoms, spending time outdoors during the day or arranging homes and workplaces to receive more sunlight may be helpful. One study found that an hour's walk in winter sunlight was as effective as two and a half hours under bright artificial light.

Side effects of phototherapy are uncommon. Some patients complain of irritability, eyestrain, headaches, or hyperactivity. No evidence has been produced of long-term adverse effects, however.

After consulting with your physician about the best treatment for you, the following suggestions may help you better manage SAD:

- Increase the amount of light in your home. Open blinds, add skylights, and trim tree branches that block sunlight.
- Walk outdoors on sunny days, even during winter.
- Exercise regularly. Physical exercise helps relieve stress and anxiety, which can accentuate SAD. Being more fit can make you feel better about yourself.
- Learn ways to better manage stress.
- If possible, take winter vacations in sunny, warm locations.

SAD IS REAL

Remember, for most people, emotional ups and downs are normal at any time of year and are not necessarily a cause for concern. However, it's important to talk to a trusted adult if you think you may be experiencing the severe symptoms of SAD. SAD is not just "all in your imagination" and, with a doctor's help, there are ways that you can feel better.

See also: Depression, Symptoms of

FURTHER READING

Rosenthal, Norman. *Winter Blues Seasonal Affective Disorder—What It Is and How to Overcome It,* Revised Edition. New York: Guilford Press, 2009.

■ SOCIAL ANXIETY DISORDER
See: Phobias

■ SOCIAL COSTS OF ANXIETY AND DEPRESSION

The costs to society of the mental disorders known as anxiety and depression. When you see the word *cost,* you probably think about money. People spend significant amounts of money each year helping or supporting people with mental disorders. Those same disorders also have large social costs—including suffering, social exclusion, disability, and poor quality of life.

Individuals and families are not the only ones to pay a price when a loved one is suffering from anxiety or depression. Society also bears some of the financial and social costs. The direct and indirect costs of mental and substance abuse disorders in the United States total more than $273 billion a year, according to the American Psychiatric Association.

DIRECT COSTS

According to a study published in the *Journal of Clinical Psychiatry,* anxiety disorders cost the United States more than $42 billion in medical costs each year. The Anxiety Disorders Association of America (2009) reports that nearly $23 billion of those costs are a result of repeat visits to doctors and hospitals because of difficulties in diagnosing anxiety disorders. Twenty percent of the doctor visits are related to **panic attacks.** People with anxiety disorders are three to five times more likely to go to the doctor and six times more likely to be hospitalized for psychiatric disorders than those who do not have the disorder. Doctors do not always connect physical symptoms with the mental disorders that may be causing them. If a doctor treats those physical symptoms—such as headaches, heavy perspiration, or stomach upset—without addressing the underlying causes, recovery is unlikely.

The World Health Organization (2009) reported that depressive disorders rank fourth in the cost of disease worldwide. These disorders are expected to rank second by 2020, behind ischemic (reduced blood supply) heart disease but ahead of all others.

The National Alliance on Mental Illness reports that the cost of untreated mental illness in the United States is $100 billion every year. In Canada, the cost is $33 billion a year in lost productivity and absenteeism.

INDIRECT COSTS

Indirect costs are costs associated with the inability of a person who is suffering from a disease to function as he or she did before the onset of the disorder. There are substantial indirect costs associated with both depression and anxiety disorders. These costs affect individuals, families, and the larger community.

On an individual level, relationships may suffer. Depressed people and those with certain anxiety disorders, such as **obsessive-compulsive disorder** or **social anxiety disorder,** often find it difficult to develop and maintain relationships. Participating in a relationship—a friendship, romance, or family relationship—requires spending time with others. A symptom of depression and many anxiety disorders is the desire to isolate oneself and spend time alone, making it difficult to maintain the connections needed to form and maintain positive, healthy relationships. Mood swings may also hamper communication. A person who is depressed or anxious may be constantly irritable or sullen; he or she may simply not have energy to devote to friends and family.

People with mental disorders may also have difficulty finding or keeping a job. They may also be at great risk of becoming involved in criminal activity and serious accidents. According to the Office of Juvenile Justice and Delinquency Prevention (2000), each year at least one out of every five young people in the juvenile justice system has serious mental health problems.

In 2009, a group of experts concluded that mental illness, in addition to substance abuse and behavioral problems among children and young adults, costs the United States $247 billion a year in treatment and lost productivity. The panel, set up by the National Research Council and Institute of Medicine, studied the financial toll caused by depression, anxiety disorders, and schizophrenia, as well as by drug and alcohol abuse and behavioral problems by people up to age 24. The $247 billion figure did not include the cost of criminal justice proceedings, education, workplace disruption, and social welfare spending. The panel said those numbers would add billions of dollars more to the price the country pays.

SCHOOL AND WORK PERFORMANCE

Depression and anxiety disorders often lead to problems at school and work. The symptoms of depression and anxiety can leave a person with so little energy that their work suffers. Those who experience

DID YOU KNOW?

Employees Experiencing Depression

At any one time, one employee in 20 is experiencing depression.

Source: National Institute of Mental Health, 2001.

anxiety or depression may also have difficulties with concentration, memory, and decision-making. The inability to concentrate fully or make decisions can lead to serious—and sometimes expensive— mistakes, particularly for those who handle dangerous equipment or make quick decisions as part of their job.

Depression and anxiety have costs not only for those suffering from the illnesses but also for those who care for them. When an employee or colleague has a family member who suffers from depression or anxiety, he or she may have trouble getting to work regularly because of the need to deal with problems at home. Caring for someone with depression or anxiety can also affect concentration and mood.

SUBSTANCE ABUSE

According to the Substance Abuse and Mental Health Services Administration, in 2007 about 21.1 percent of Americans age 18 to 25 needed treatment for alcohol (17.2 percent) or illicit drug use (8.4 percent). In addition, 4.4 percent of people in that age group needed treatment for both alcohol and illicit drug use. Less than 7.0 percent of the young adults who needed drug and alcohol treatment received that therapy. Ninety-six percent of the young adults who needed treatment said they did not see the need for therapy. Less than one-third who needed treatment actually attempted to obtain it.

After using drugs or alcohol, many people suffering from anxiety and depression behave recklessly and put themselves in serious danger. The National Center for Health Statistics reported the top three causes of death for 15- to 24-year-olds were automobile crashes, homicide, and suicide. Alcohol was a leading factor in all three.

The abuse of drugs and alcohol by people with depression or anxiety disorders has both financial and social costs to businesses, schools, and communities. Attendance at school may slide because of truancy (skipping school) due to drug or alcohol use. Conflicts with coworkers or fellow students may increase because of the moodiness that is a symptom of depression, anxiety disorders, and substance abuse. A study by the JSI Research and Training Institute (1998) showed that one in five workers report that they have had to work harder, redo work, cover for a coworker, or been exposed to danger or even injured as a result a fellow employee's drinking. Substance Abuse and Mental Health Services Administration (1998) reported that substance abusers were five times more likely to file worker's compensation claims than their drug-free coworkers. Other costs, such as low morale and high absentee rates due to illness, are less obvious costs, but the effects are equally harmful.

FAMILY AND COMMUNITY DYSFUNCTION

When someone suffers from a mental disorder such as depression or an anxiety disorder, the whole family is affected. If a brother, sister, father, mother, or other close relative has depression or an anxiety disorder, the rest of the family may alter behavior to try to accommodate the needs of the ill person.

The U.S. Department of Justice's Bureau of Justice Statistics reports that the nation's prison system has become a warehouse for the mentally ill. The department says that 64 percent of local jail inmates, 56 percent of state prisoners, and 45 percent of federal prisoners have symptoms of serious mental illnesses. The figures are much worse than previously thought. Estimates had previously put the total number of inmates with mental health issues at 20 percent of the prison population.

Most inmates with mental disorders do not receive treatment while they are in prison. As a result, they are still suffering from those disorders when they leave jail and may repeat their illegal behaviors, costing the community even more money. In fact, CJMHCP (2002) reported that **recidivism** (repetition of criminal behavior) rates for inmates with mental illness was over 70 percent in some areas.

Fact Or Fiction?

Having a phobia isn't serious. It's not as though I'll lose friends because of it.

The Facts: Even a simple phobia like a fear of dogs can be problematic. For example, suppose a good friend invites you to his or her house. You'd like to go, but your friend owns a dog. If your friend does not understand how powerful phobias are, he or she may feel slighted if you refuse to visit. Other phobias can also come between friends, especially when the disorder is not taken seriously. If you are suffering from a phobia, explain to your friends that you have a disorder and don't mean to be rude. A good friend will understand. You have no reason to be embarrassed.

COSTS IN PERSPECTIVE

The costs of depression and anxiety disorders are both financial and social. On a social level, people who know and care about depressed or anxious people are affected by the disorder. Financially, the costs impact both the national and global economy, according to the World Health Organization. These significant costs indicate that depression and anxiety are serious disorders. Fortunately, they are also treatable. Most people with depression or anxiety disorders who get professional help are able to contribute fully to society.

See also: Codependency; Depression and Substance Abuse

FURTHER READING

Sartorius, Norman. *Reducing the Stigma of Mental Illness: A Report From a Global Association.* New York: Cambridge University Press, 2005.

■ SUICIDE AND DEPRESSION

Suicide is the act of taking one's own life as the result of experiencing long periods of hopelessness or unhappiness. Most people experience short periods of sadness and even despair. Loss, rejection, and disappointment are a part of life, and sadness and pain are normal reactions. However, for some people the pain is so intense that they feel completely hopeless. Some have suicidal thoughts—all they can think about is death. If people don't speak openly about such thoughts, they may come to believe that suicide is the only way to end their pain. They are wrong.

Suicide is a hard subject for some people to discuss. Regardless of the sensitivity of the subject, suicide is a form of violence, and thoughts of suicide are something people have to talk and think about if they want to find answers for people who have lost all hope.

According to the National Institute of Mental Health (NIMH), many people who contemplate suicide—at least 90 percent—suffer from **mental disorders**. A mental disorder is an illness that alters or changes thinking, mood, or behavior. These changes often cause emotional pain. Depression and **bipolar disorder** (a mental disorder that shifts from periods of depression to periods of extreme excitement, or **mania**) are both painful disorders if left untreated.

Although modern treatments for mental disorders are effective, there is no "one size fits all" treatment. Mental health professions have a variety of treatments that can help those who contemplate suicide. Getting that help is essential.

"CLUSTER" SUICIDES"

"Cluster" suicides are multiple suicides that occur in a particular place within a defined period of time. Researchers believe that one death may prompt the others in much the way a contagious disease may spread through a community. Adolescents are particularly prone to "cluster" suicides.

The media covers these tragedies so intensely that it is easy to believe that "cluster" suicides and even group suicides are common. If fact, they are not. The Centers for Disease Control and Prevention reported in 2009 that suicide pacts are relatively rare. Suicide clusters in general account for no more than 1 to 5 percent of all suicides by young people.

BIPOLAR DISORDER AND SUICIDE

According to the American Foundation for Suicide Prevention (AFSP), patients suffering from depression and bipolar disorder are far more likely to take their own lives than individuals in any other psychiatric or medical risk group. The AFSP also reports that 25 to 50 percent of bipolar people attempt suicide at least once. Despite these sobering facts, treatments for people with depressive disorder are successful in alleviating symptoms over 80 percent of the time (AFSP).

Because both manic and depressive episodes can have serious consequences, the Depression and Bipolar Support Alliance recommends that people suffering with bipolar disorder develop a plan for dealing with a severe manic or depressive episode. The plan should be shared with a trusted family member and/or friend. It might include having a friend or relation contact the doctor, take control of credit cards and car keys, and/or increase contact with family or friends until the severe episode has passed.

Those who have a bipolar disorder, like all people, have good and bad days. Being in a bad mood one day is not necessarily a sign of an upcoming severe episode. Working with a professional doctor or therapist can help differentiate between a normal mood swing and a manic or depressive episode.

CAUSES OF SUICIDE

The reasons for suicide are unpredictable. When faced with a major disappointment, rejection, or loss, most people react with sadness or frustration. Others may respond with anger that seems out of proportion to the event. Still others may find the disappointment unbearable and turn to thoughts of suicide in the belief that the sadness and frustration will never end. Among the factors that may prompt someone to consider suicide are family turmoil, access to deadly suicide methods (Johns Hopkins Bloomberg School of Public Health reported in 2005 that 52 percent of all suicides are death by a firearm), a history of physical or sexual abuse, the loss of a friend or loved one, social isolation, loneliness, or alcohol or drug use. Research suggests that suicide is not **hereditary**. It does not "run in the family."

People can be especially susceptible to suicidal thoughts during their teen years. Adolescents experience dramatic biochemical changes. Sudden mood swings are common, and some feelings seem to have no apparent reason. As their sexuality emerges, teens are faced with new experiences, feelings, and challenges. These sometimes disorienting changes can be complicated by substance use and abuse.

The teen years are also often filled with intensive self-examination. Young people often ask themselves, "Who am I?" and "Why don't I fit in?" These questions can lead some people into darkness and despair, especially if they are already experiencing depression or other mental disorders.

Another element that makes being a teenager especially difficult is the realization that one is about to become an adult. As a child, one feels like an extension of his or her parents. As an adolescent, one sees once-respected adults now as authority figures who seem to want the teenager to stay a child forever. Many wish their parents would do more than just tell them what they can't do. These changes in the relationship between teenagers and their parents can lead to heated discussions and disagreements that are often exacerbated by a lack of good communication. Hurt feelings on both sides are common and can lead to serious emotional distress—and depression.

Some young people are idealistic. They have high moral and ethical standards that they would like everyone to live up to. Life is not perfect. Bad things happen. People are not perfect either. They make mistakes. Those who are particularly idealistic may be disturbed or disappointed by life's ups and downs.

Community loss—the tragedy of September 11, the loss of the Columbia shuttle, the wars in Afghanistan and Iraq—can have devastating effects. Especially if a person is already feeling things are hopeless, it's easy to see international, national, or local tragedies as evidence that nothing and no one is safe.

TEENAGERS

Suicide is a risk for anyone, especially those with mental disorders like depression or anxiety. It is a particular danger for teens. In fact, according to the Centers for Disease Control and Prevention, suicide is the third leading cause of death among 15- to 24-year-olds, behind unintentional injury and homicide. The National Strategy for Suicide Prevention reported in 1999 that more young adults died as a result of suicide than cancer, heart disease, HIV/AIDS, stroke, pneumonia, influenza, and chronic lung disease combined.

According to government statistics, about 20 percent of U.S. teens will experience some sort of depression before they reach adulthood. In addition, between 10 to 15 percent of teenagers exhibit some symptoms of depression at any one time, while 5 percent suffer from major bouts of depression. Moreover, 8.3 percent of teens will be depressed for a year at a time, compared to 5.3 percent of the general population.

Most teens will suffer from more than one episode of depression, while 20 to 40 percent will have more than one episode within two years. Statistics show that 70 percent of teens will have more than one episode of depression before adulthood. Each episode generally lasts for about eight months.

SENIOR CITIZENS

Young people are not the only group at risk for suicide. Senior citizens are at even greater risk. According to a 2003 report by NIMH, although senior citizens comprise only 13 percent of the population, people age 65 and older accounted for 18 percent of all suicide deaths in the United States in 2000. Among the highest rates (when catego-

DID YOU KNOW?

A Day of Remembrance

Each year, the Saturday before Thanksgiving is National Survivors of Suicide Day.

Source: American Foundation for Suicide Prevention.

rized by gender and race) were white men age 85 and older: 59 deaths per 100,000 persons in 2000, more than five times the national U.S. rate of 10.6 per 100,000.

Social isolation may contribute to many of the suicides among seniors. A suicidal crisis for seniors often follows being widowed, the death of a friend or relative, living alone, or anticipation of placement in a nursing home. As with younger people, suicide among the elderly is associated with depression, alcoholism, chronic medical illness, and having access to firearms. People who are depressed—young and old—should not use alcohol or drugs or have access to firearms. The National Strategy for Suicide Prevention (1998) reported that death by firearms was the most common method of suicide (71 percent) among persons age 65 years and older.

GENDER DIFFERENCES

Gender plays a role in suicide attempts and suicide. The NIMH reported that suicide was the seventh-leading cause of death for males and the 16th-leading cause of death for females in 2007. More than four times as many men as women die by suicide, according to the NIMH, although women report attempting suicide during their lifetime about three times as often as men. Suicide by firearm is the most common method for both men and women, accounting for 56 percent of male suicides and 31 percent of female suicides in 2006.

There are gender differences in young people who take their own lives as well. The Centers for Disease Control and Prevention (2009) reported that among youths 15 to 19, boys were five times as likely as girls to commit suicide; among 20- to 24-year-olds, males were seven times as likely as females to commit suicide.

TEENS SPEAK

My Friend Wanted to Die

When Rosemary showed me the inside of her purse, I didn't know what to think.

"I think I'm going to take these," she said, smiling.

She took out a handful of pills and shuffled them from one hand to the next. There were all sorts of colors and shapes; they almost looked like candy.

"What will they do?" I asked, not sure what to say.

"I'll die," she said, still smiling.

I couldn't believe she was smiling. She must be kidding, I thought, although I didn't think it was very funny. I had to say so.

"That's not funny, Rosemary," I said.

"Oh, I'm not kidding," she said.

I was pretty freaked out. What was she telling me? Was she serious?

At our next class, I couldn't concentrate. Last year, the captain of our cheerleading team killed herself. No one expected it. It took a long time for things to get back to normal. The school offered special group meetings with counselors for those of us who wanted to talk about it. I remember one of the counselors, Ms. Brown, talking about how to tell if someone is suicidal. If someone talks about wanting to commit suicide, we were told to *always* take it seriously. I knew Rosemary had had some pretty big emotional ups and downs. This year has been especially tough for her. Her boyfriend broke up with her in front of everyone in the cafeteria. But I didn't think she was feeling bad enough to kill herself!

By the end of class I had thought about it enough; I knew what I had to do. I walked over to Rosemary and said, "I don't know if you were kidding or not, but knowing you may be planning to hurt yourself is too much for me to keep secret. Let's go talk to Ms. Brown together right now."

"No, I'm fine," said Rosemary.

"Well," I said, "I'm going to go talk to her. Suicide scares me, and I don't want you to die."

I went straight to Ms. Brown's office and told her what Rosemary had said. She talked to me for a while. She told me that telling her what I had learned was the right thing to do. She also told me that what Rosemary did or didn't do was not my responsibility. She said she would try to talk to her immediately.

I felt pretty weird telling on Rosemary, but the way she said, "I'll die," with a smile really scared me. I think it would have scared me even if she hadn't smiled.

Ms. Brown did talk to Rosemary and Rosemary took some time off from school. When she came back, she seemed really grounded. She came up to me and thanked me for talking to Ms. Brown.

"I didn't think anyone would take me seriously," said Rosemary, "and that was the problem. You heard me and I'm grateful."

WARNING SIGNS

If you are concerned that a friend or loved one may have thoughts of suicide, talk to him or her about it and tell an adult you trust. You shouldn't ignore what might seem like casual remarks or jokes, such as "You'll be sorry when I'm dead" or "There's no way out . . . ." Such comments, no matter how offhand they seem, may indicate serious suicidal feelings. You should take all threats seriously. You are not betraying someone's trust by trying to keep him or her alive.

Many behaviors can help you recognize the threat of suicide. Warning signs include

- severe, prolonged depression
- marked changes in personality or behavior (a sudden swing from extremely depressed to extremely happy)
- a sudden change in friends
- extreme changes in eating and sleeping habits
- decreased academic performance
- running away from home

- becoming irresponsible
- making a will or giving away prized possessions
- a suicide threat or statement indicating a desire to die
- a previous suicide attempt

These symptoms do not necessarily mean a friend or loved one is suicidal. However, if the behaviors are unusual for that person, they may be signs of trouble. If the changes are dramatic, it's especially important to speak openly with the individual about them to determine if the changes are related to depression.

Q & A

Question: My friend's mother committed suicide—how can I help my friend?

Answer: Here are a few tips to follow if you have a friend who is dealing with the aftermath of a personal loss:

- Reach out and spend time with your friend.
- Make time to talk, encourage your friend to express his or her feelings, and listen.
- Respect his or her need to spend time alone.
- Help with everyday tasks where possible—run errands, share a meal, pick up mail, care for a pet, or find another way to help.
- Don't try to offer false cheer or "fix things"; listening without judging is a powerful form of support.
- Help your friend connect with supportive resources at school or in the community.
- Encourage him or her to seek professional help.
- Take care of yourself and know your own limits.

PREVENTIVE ACTIONS

Suicide is preventable and the warning signs are treatable. If you have a friend who is thinking about suicide, discussing his or her thoughts may be a good way to be of help. However, in every case, finding professional help is essential. People who are considering suicide often are not capable of seeking the help they need, so you may need to provide them with some of the phone numbers at the end of this book. You may also want to call one of the hotlines to get advice about your friend's particular situation. Professionals can help support you, but the goal is to connect your friend with an expert.

Communication

People who are contemplating suicide feel alone and helpless. The most important thing a person can do to stop them is to talk with them openly and often. Be willing to listen without criticizing.

People who feel suicidal often want a friend, someone to listen to them, even if they seem reluctant to open up. Remember that some people do not know how to reach out for help when they need it and they may need someone to reach *in*.

A common misconception is that talking about suicide with someone who is considering it might make matters worse. In fact, bringing up the issue without expressing shock or judgment is one of the best things you can do.

Fact Or Fiction?

People who talk openly about their thoughts of suicide are not at risk of committing the act. In other words, if a friend talks about committing suicide, he or she won't actually go through with it.

The Facts: If a friend talks about committing suicide in any way, he or she is asking for help. It is important to let your friend know that you are there for him or her. It is also important that you contact a teacher, parent, or other adult you trust to get help for your friend.

Crisis

If the threat is immediate—if a friend tells you that he or she is going to commit suicide soon—don't leave him or her alone and don't try to argue with him or her. Ask questions like "Have you thought about how you'll do it?" and "Have you decided when or where?" If the person has a defined plan and an easily available method of suicide (such as a gun or pills), then the risk of suicide is severe. You should immediately take your friend to a hospital emergency room or call 911.

Remember, even the most severely depressed person has mixed feelings about death. Most people don't want to die—they just want the pain to stop. Those who threaten suicide have lost sight of the fact that the impulse to "end it all" *does not last forever.*

RECOVERY

Professional treatment for the mental disorders associated with suicidal thoughts can be extraordinarily successful. The belief that once a person is suicidal he or she is forever suicidal is a myth. The truth is that most people remain suicidal for only a limited time—though the feeling can seem unending!

Still, it is important to be wary. After someone has received treatment and says he or she is feeling better, don't automatically believe it. Sometimes people find it easier to put on a happy face to avoid seeming crazy or weird. According to the organization Suicide Awareness/ Voices of Education (2003), a number of people commit suicide just as they seem to be getting better, perhaps because they did not have the energy to kill themselves when they were extremely depressed but now have just enough energy to go through with their plan.

WHAT TO DO IF YOU FEEL SUICIDAL

If you feel suicidal, do not drink alcohol or use drugs. Get help now—not later. Talk to a trusted adult, teacher, counselor, or member of the clergy. Call 911 or 1-800-SUICIDE, or check in your phone book for the number of a suicide crisis center. Trained volunteers and professional counselors staff these centers. They can help callers identify their problems, explore options, and develop a plan of action. These hotlines also provide referrals to community-based services and support groups. Life may seem bad sometimes, but those times don't last forever. Suicide doesn't have to be the answer. There are many other solutions. Asking for help can make you feel better.

Caring people who understand what you're feeling want to help you, not judge you. You don't need to be ashamed of your feelings; many teenagers feel the same way. Remember, no matter how serious the problem, there is always hope.

See also: Anxiety Disorders; Anxiety Disorders, Symptoms of; Depression, Causes of; Depression, Symptoms of; Gender and Depression;

Media and Anxiety and Depression, The; Morbidity and Mortality; Rehabilitation and Treatment of Depression; Resiliency

FURTHER READING

De Leo, D., ed., et al. *Attempted Suicide: A Handbook of Treatment, Theory, and Recent Findings.* Cambridge, Mass.: Hogrefe & Huber, 2004.

Henden, John. *Preventing Suicide: The Solution Focused Approach.* New York: Wiley, 2008.

■ TREATMENT OF ANXIETY DISORDERS

Treatment to restore to a healthy state from an illness such as an anxiety disorder or depression, usually with medication, therapy, or a combination of the two. Anxiety disorders are mental disorders that cause similar to fear symptoms. They are among the most treatable of all mental illnesses. Nearly all of those who receive treatment feel better, even though they may not be completely "cured." Like many other mental illnesses, rehabilitation for anxiety disorders usually includes medication, therapy, or a combination of the two.

Researchers in 2008 found that a combination of a commonly prescribed antidepressant and a specialized type of talk therapy worked well in treating children with anxiety disorders. Researchers reported that the anxiety levels of 81 percent of children, ages seven to 17, who took the antidepressant Zoloft while participating in 14 sessions of cognitive behavioral therapy improved significantly over those children who took only Zoloft or participated in just the therapy sessions. Researchers found that 60 percent of the children who participated in therapy got better. In addition, 55 percent in the Zoloft-only group improved, while only 24 percent in a group who only took a **placebo** got better.

Recovering from anxiety disorders means successfully challenging "cognitive distortions." Cognitive distortions are the mistaken beliefs people have about themselves. For example, stress affects everyone and is everywhere, but doubting one's ability to manage the stress may lead to anxiety. There is a theory about the cause of anxiety based on cognitive distortions, aptly named the cognitive distortions theory. According to this theory, anxiety often results from errors in thinking, such as jumping to conclusions, exaggerating the negative, and ignoring the positive. Such thinking may lead one to a gloomy view of oneself, the world, and one's future.

INDIVIDUAL PSYCHOTHERAPY AND COUNSELING

There are nearly 200 psychotherapy techniques used by mental health professionals. Anxiety is usually treated with **individual therapy,** which is one kind of psychotherapy. In individual therapy—often referred to as counseling—a client meets one-on-one with a therapist. However, in a strict sense, psychotherapy differs from counseling.

Psychotherapy involves an examination of one's behaviors. The client is expected to talk about those behaviors in an effort to change them. A behavior can be an action, a thought, a statement, a memory, a sensation, or an emotion. Changing behaviors is hard work.

Rather than talking about behaviors, a counselor provides or helps individuals create activities that are likely to bring about changes—much the way exercise does. Counseling usually results in a realization, a plan, or a decision.

Both psychotherapy and counseling may be successful in reducing anxiety. Both methods involve talking with a professional therapist and require dedication and **introspection,** a self-examination of feelings, thoughts, and motives. Both individual therapy and counseling are often referred to as "talk therapy," because of their reliance on conversations between a patient and a professional therapist.

People who experience anxiety often have poor planning skills, high stress levels, and difficulty relaxing. Therapists can help them in many ways, especially by teaching relaxation skills.

DRUG THERAPY

Medication can help relieve symptoms, but there is no simple cure. Today people have access to more medications that effectively treat anxiety disorders than ever before. The same **antidepressants** used to treat depression are often useful in treating anxiety disorders. Other medications (described in the following pages) used to treat anxiety include benzodiazepines, and, less commonly, beta-blockers.

There are several categories of antidepressants that have proved effective in the treatment of anxiety disorders. The most recently developed and most commonly used group are the selective serotonin reuptake inhibitors, or SSRIs. SSRIs act on a chemical called **serotonin** that helps the brain regulate mood and emotions.

Serotonin levels have been linked to anxiety, depression, and migraine headaches. In people who do not suffer from anxiety disorder, serotonin moves between nerve cells in the brain according to a specific pattern. Serotonin is released into the space between the "sending" nerve cells and the "receiving" nerve cells. When serotonin is received on the surface of the "receiving cell," it stimulates or activates serotonin receptors. Stimulation of these receptors generates an impulse and allows a message to move forward. When serotonin is released from a "sending" nerve cell, a serotonin **uptake pump** reabsorbs some of it. A person who suffers from an anxiety disorder may have a problem balancing serotonin levels. By blocking the serotonin uptake pump, SSRIs increase the amount of active serotonin that can be delivered to a "receiving" nerve cell, and this may help message transmission return to normal. To summarize, SSRIs treat anxiety by "selectively" blocking the reuptake of serotonin.

SSRIs tend to have fewer side effects than older antidepressants. Side effects may include nausea or agitation when first taking the medication, but the effects generally lessen over time. Some people also experience sexual difficulties when taking some of these medications. An adjustment in dosage or a switch to another SSRI usually corrects these problems.

Tricyclics have been prescribed for many more years than SSRIs and their use in treating anxiety disorders has been more widely studied. For anxiety disorders other than obsessive-compulsive disorder, they are as effective as the SSRIs. However, many doctors and people with anxiety disorders prefer SSRIs, because tricyclics may cause dizziness, drowsiness, dry mouth, and weight gain.

The oldest group of antidepressants are the **monoamine oxidase inhibitors,** or MAOIs. People who take MAOIs are put on a restrictive diet because these medications can interact with foods and beverages, including cheese and red wine, that contain a chemical called tyramine. MAOIs also interact with some other medications, including SSRIs. Interactions between MAOIs and other substances can cause dangerous elevations in blood pressure or other potentially life-threatening reactions.

Another group of medications used to treat anxiety are the benzodiazepines. One of the benefits of these drugs is that they can relieve symptoms within a short time. They have relatively few side effects. Drowsiness and loss of coordination are the most common effects; fatigue and mental slowing, or confusion, can also occur. These effects make it dangerous for people taking benzodiazepines to drive or operate some machinery.

Benzodiazepines are also referred to as minor tranquilizers. They work by slowing down the activity of the central nervous system. They slow the messages between the brain and the body, including physical, mental, and emotional responses. Like alcohol, they are depressants.

More often used to treat heart patients, beta-blockers treat anxiety by reducing the body's response to **adrenaline**. Adrenaline is a chemical that is naturally produced in response to fear. Beta-blockers are used to calm anxiety symptoms such as shaking, palpitations, and excessive perspiration. They also reduce blood pressure and slow the heartbeat. Beta-blockers are fast acting and non-habit-forming, but should not be taken by people with other preexisting medical conditions such as diabetes or asthma.

INPATIENT TREATMENT

Anxiety disorders are usually treated through individual therapy on an outpatient basis. Treatment given to someone residing in a healthcare facility is called **inpatient treatment**. If the anxiety disorder is severely disabling, inpatient treatment may be appropriate.

Q & A

Question: If I put myself in stressful situations on purpose, will I get over my anxiety?

Answer: If you seek out difficult situations as a cure for anxiety, you are almost guaranteed to fail. It is more likely that the forced situations will cause you embarrassment and further anxiety. It is important to begin the recovery process more gradually and work up to more and more stressful social situations. You are also more likely to have more success if you talk with a therapist as you face situations that cause you anxiety.

ALTERNATIVE TREATMENTS

In addition to the standard treatments for anxiety disorders—therapy and medication—some people seek alternative treatments. "Medications and psychotherapy are still the mainstays when it comes to treating . . . anxiety," says Ronald Glick, the medical director of the Center for Complementary Medicine at the University of Pittsburgh Medical Center-Shadyside and professor of psychiatry at the University of Pittsburgh School of Medicine. "But alternative therapies can help. It depends on what you expect from them."

Some symptoms of anxiety and depression may be relieved by such practices as

- relaxation techniques—deep breathing, meditation, prayer, or hypnosis
- exercise—yoga, Pilates, even walking 15 minutes a day
- creative arts therapies—using dance, music, art, drama as outlets for emotional expression

Many alternative treatments rely on the body's energy for healing. The energy may be described in different ways. For example, exercise typical in the United States such as running or walking oxygenates the blood and can increase the level of relaxing endorphins in the body. Chinese-based acupuncture describes the flow of the body's "life-force," or chi, as the healing energy activated or influenced by the acupuncture treatments.

It is important for people with troublesome anxiety disorders to receive professional help. An alternative therapy should not be used as a replacement for a consultation with a physician. People who rely on alternatives too much—who don't get treatment that is proven to be effective—can slip into a more serious and potentially dangerous anxiety disorder before they realize it.

ANXIETY DISORDERS ARE TREATABLE

Without treatment, anxiety disorders can make it difficult to go to school, visit friends, or just leave the house. Useful professional help comes in different forms. Some people rely on talk therapy such as psychotherapy or counseling. Others may work with a professional to treat their disorder with medication. Anxiety disorders are treatable— there is no need to suffer.

See also: Anxiety Disorders, Common Types; Anxiety Disorders, Symptoms of

FURTHER READING

Hollander, Eric, and Daphne Simeon. *Concise Guide to Anxiety Disorders.* Arlington, Va.: American Psychiatric Publishing, Incorporated, 2002.

DiTomasso, Robert A., and Elizabeth A. Gosch, *Comparative Treatments for Anxiety Disorders.* New York: Springer Publishing Co., 2002.

■ TREATMENT OF DEPRESSION

Restoring to a healthy state through various therapies from a mental disorder caused by a chemical imbalance in the brain. The treatment of a person with depression by medication, by **psychotherapy,** or with a combination of the two is often referred to as rehabilitation. Depression, characterized by feelings of sadness and a general loss of interest in life, involves a change in chemicals in the brain. People with depression cannot "just snap out of it." However, most people with depression can be successfully treated. Because depression can be caused by various medical illnesses and medications, people with symptoms of depression should have a physical exam before treatment begins.

Until the twentieth century, most people experiencing depression were neither diagnosed nor treated. In most cases, family provided what little care was available. Research over the past few decades has dramatically increased the range of possibilities for treating depression.

Fact Or Fiction?

The medications used to treat depression turn people into drug addicts.

The Facts: Antidepressants have come a long way in the past 20 years. They used to have many serious side effects, such as dry mouth and dizziness. Many of the new antidepressants work as well as the older ones but have many fewer side effects. Antidepressants are not addictive.

DRUG THERAPY

Antidepressants are medications that prevent or relieve depression. Antidepressants are usually prescribed for serious depressions, but they can also be helpful for milder cases. Antidepressants are not "uppers" or stimulants. Instead they remove or reduce the symptoms of depression and help people feel the way they did before they became depressed.

Prescription drugs

While some people feel better within a week of starting an antidepressant, many find they do not experience the beneficial effects until two to four weeks after beginning the medication. Still others experience an even more delayed reaction to the medication; they may not see benefits for months.

There are several categories of effective antidepressants. The most commonly used group are the **selective serotonin reuptake inhibitors,** or SSRIs. SSRIs, which include Prozac (fluoxetine) and Zoloft (sertraline), act on a chemical called **serotonin** that helps the brain communicate with itself through nerve cells.

To send a message, a "sending" nerve cell releases a certain amount of serotonin, which then moves toward a "receiving" nerve cell. Through this process, the "sending" cell reabsorbs some of the serotonin through an **uptake pump,** which is how the brain makes sure that the "receiving" cell gets just the right amount of serotonin to stimulate the receptors in that cell, generate an impulse, and allow the message to move forward.

When a person suffers from depression, the uptake pump may be removing too much serotonin. The resulting imbalance can trigger an anxiety disorder, depression, or even migraine headaches. By blocking the serotonin uptake pump, SSRIs increase the amount of active serotonin that can be delivered to the "receiving" nerve cell, which may help message transmission return to normal.

SSRIs tend to have fewer side effects than other antidepressants. Side effects may include nausea or agitation when first taking the medication, but the effects generally disappear over time. Some people also experience sexual difficulties when taking some of these medications. An adjustment in dosage or a switch to another SSRI or a different type of antidepressant usually corrects these problems.

Tricyclics have been around longer than SSRIs and have been more widely studied as a treatment for depression. Many doctors and their patients prefer the SSRIs, because the tricyclics may cause dizziness, drowsiness, dry mouth, and weight gain. Tricyclics prescribed to treat depression include imipramine and amitriptyline.

The oldest group of antidepressants are the **monoamine oxidase inhibitors,** or MAOIs. Nardil (phenelzine) and Parnate (tranylcypromine) are two MAOIs often used to treat depression. People who take MAOIs must follow a restrictive diet, because these medications interact with foods and beverages, including cheese and red wine, that contain the chemical tyramine. MAOIs also interact with some other medications, including SSRIs. Interactions between MAOIs and other substances can cause a dangerous rise in blood pressure and other potentially life-threatening reactions.

Herbal remedies

According to a 2002 report in the *Journal of the American Medical Association* some people claim that an herbal supplement, known as *Hypericum* or Saint-John's-wort, has antidepressant properties. However, results from the first large-scale, controlled study of the herb, funded in part by NIMH, revealed that it was no more effective in treating depression of moderate severity than a placebo—a "sugar pill" with no medicinal value. More research is needed to determine the role of Saint-John's-wort in managing less severe forms of depression. Using herbal remedies can be dangerous. There is evidence, for example, that taking Saint-John's-wort can reduce the effectiveness of certain medications. People should always discuss its use—or that of any other herbal or natural supplement—with their doctor before trying it.

Rates

IMS Health, a marketing research company, reports that that doctors handed out 232.7 million prescriptions for antidepressants in 2007, more than any other type of drug. Moreover, the U.S. sales of these drugs totaled $11.9 billion in 2007. According to IMS Health, the sales of antidepressants worldwide jumped 0.6 percent in 2008 to $20.3 billion.

Drug companies such as Wyeth, Eli Lilly, Forest Laboratories, GlaxoSmithKline, Pfizer, and Merck are among the big players in the antidepressant marketplace. For example, Wyeth's Effexor accounted for $3.93 billion in U.S. sales in 2008. The sales of Eli Lilly's Cymbalta grew the fastest of all antidepressants, from $2.1 billion in 2007 to $2.7 billion in 2008.

TEENS SPEAK

Until I Faced My Addictions, I Couldn't Deal with My Depression

I was in therapy for a long time before I started to deal with my addictions. In fact, I was diagnosed with depression a year before I started to get help for my substance abuse problems. I think my therapist didn't see the problem because I was in so much denial I just never talked about my drinking.

This was more dangerous than I realized. I didn't know that the antidepressants I was prescribed didn't interact well with alcohol. I started experiencing blackouts a lot more often—I'd wake up and realize I couldn't remember what I'd done after I started drinking the night before. Although the medication and the therapy did help some—I was able to get out of bed most mornings—I really didn't feel much better. I was walking around in a daze. I didn't think I could be suffering from addiction because everyone around me partied so much more than I did.

But when I found myself with no more friends after getting into drunken fights with everyone I knew and loved, I started to wonder what was wrong. I asked my therapist if there could be something wrong besides my depression. She asked me a lot of questions. I finally told her how I had lost friends because I was drunk. I also told her how I would do things when I was drunk that I would never do when I was sober. I felt like I turned into someone else when I was intoxicated. I used to like that feeling, but it was getting me into more and more trouble.

My therapist and I agreed that I would go to a 12–step group meeting to learn more about alcoholism and addiction. I called the local number for Alcoholics Anonymous and a woman took me to a meeting the next day.

Soon after I got sober, the therapy and medication for my depression worked in ways they never had before. I found myself. I got my personality back and started living my life the way I had wanted to for so long. If I hadn't faced my alcoholism, I would have never healed my depression.

INDIVIDUAL PSYCHOTHERAPY AND COUNSELING

Depression is usually treated with **individual therapy,** which is one type of psychotherapy. In individual therapy, a client meets alone with a therapist. In some ways psychotherapy is similar to counseling, but there are important differences. Psychotherapy involves the examination of one's behaviors. It takes hard work to change many of those behaviors by talking about them. Instead of encouraging clients to talk about their behaviors, counseling provides or helps individual clients create activities that bring about change—in much the way that exercises can change the body.

Both psychotherapy and counseling may be successful in reducing depression. Both methods involve discussion with a professional therapist and require introspection. **Introspection** is self-examination of one's feelings, thoughts, and motives.

Individual therapy and counseling are often referred to as "talk therapy" because of their reliance on conversations between a patient and a professional therapist. These conversations help individuals deal with their depression. Therapy can help not only improve self-esteem but also repair relationships that have suffered as a result of the depression. Therapy may also be a source of knowledge about mental disorders, what they are, how they affect the sufferer, and how therapy may help treat the illnesses.

One study published in 2006 in the *American Journal of Psychiatry* reported that patients with chronic depression are rarely helped by antidepressants. However, another study, published at the same time, reported that medication provided complete relief for 30 percent of patients who have recurrent bouts of depression, while only half saw no improvement whatsoever.

GROUP THERAPY

Group therapy is a form of psychotherapy involving at least two patients and a therapist. Participants are encouraged to analyze their own and each other's problems. Group therapy has many of the same goals as individual therapy but relies on advice, feedback, and support from others in the group to help participants learn how to deal with problems. Unlike a support group, which may be led by peers or laypersons, professionals always lead group therapy sessions.

Group sessions may take place in a private practice, community mental health center, hospital, or other professional setting. In most cases, group members did not know each other before meeting for therapy. Those who generally benefit most from these sessions are individuals who are willing to share personal experiences, thoughts, and feelings with a group and listen to other people's fears and frustrations, instead of focusing solely on their own. Often participants discover that their past experiences are helpful to other members.

FAMILY THERAPY

Family therapy can be useful in helping spouses, parents, and children work together to overcome depression and its effects. Whether one member of the family is depressed or more than one member, family therapy can be a useful tool. Instead of focusing on the

---

DID YOU KNOW?

Generic and Common Brand Names for Some Popular SSRI Medications

Brand Name	Generic Name
Prozac	fluoxetine
Zoloft	sertraline
Paxil	paroxetine
Luvox	fluvoxamine
Celexa	citalopram

Source: International Coalition for Drug Awareness.

individual, family therapy focuses on interactions among family members.

A family may decide to go to therapy together if members are having problems that interfere with the way the family functions or if individual therapy doesn't seem to be helping. The goal is to resolve the problems as quickly and effectively as possible.

INPATIENT TREATMENT

Some people suffering from depression may need to stay in a hospital or treatment center as part of their recovery. A team of professionals generally provides **inpatient treatment.** The therapists work with family members to help find therapies for both the hospital stay and the period after discharge. Patients may actively participate in creating their treatment plan.

TYPES OF THERAPY

Though there are hundreds of forms of therapy, two forms of psychotherapy that have been very effective in dealing with depression are **cognitive behavior therapy** and **interpersonal therapy.**

Cognitive behavior therapy

Cognitive behavior therapy (CBT) is based on the idea that "you are what you think." This type of therapy maintains that pessimistic thoughts contribute to depression. According to this theory, people experiencing depression often have negative views of

- themselves. They view themselves as worthless, inadequate, helpless, unlovable, and deficient.
- their environment. They see it as overwhelming, unsupportive, and filled with obstacles.
- the future. They regard it as hopeless.

The goal of CBT is to replace negative thoughts with more positive, realistic perceptions. Participants learn to recognize depressive reactions and associated thoughts, usually by keeping a journal of their ideas and responses. The patient and the therapist then develop ways to challenge these negative reactions and thoughts through homework assignments, such as reading about depression or communicating with others. The process helps individuals learn how to replace negative responses with more positive ones.

Interpersonal therapy

Interpersonal therapy focuses on relationships as a way of understanding and overcoming depression. The goal of interpersonal therapy is to improve relationship and communication skills and boost self-esteem. Interpersonal therapy typically explores four areas:

- unresolved grief,
- conflicts or disputes with others,
- transitions from one social role to another,
- difficulties with interpersonal or people skills.

Like cognitive behavior therapy, interpersonal therapy is short-term. Interpersonal therapy has three phases of treatment. In its initial phase, the goal is to identify problem areas. In the middle phase, the focus is on dealing with and resolving one or more key issues. In the final phase, the therapist and the client work on ways of ending therapy.

Long-term therapy

Many people who are depressed benefit most from individual sessions with a therapist, but some find a group setting more helpful. They may attend therapy sessions with their spouse or family. Group, couples, and family therapy may be based on cognitive behavior strategies, interpersonal techniques, or a combination of these and other therapies.

The goal of long-term therapy is to identify and change patterns of behavior that increase a person's risk of depression. Individuals most likely to benefit from long-term therapy are those whose depression is accompanied by another mental illness, such as an anxiety disorder, an eating disorder, substance abuse, a personality disorder, or by persistently painful or costly patterns of behavior.

ALTERNATIVE THERAPIES

In addition to the standard treatments for depression—therapy and medication—some people seek alternative treatments. Many alternative treatments rely on the body's energy. The energy may be described in different ways. For example, exercise typical in the United States such as running or walking oxygenates the blood and can increase the level of endorphins in the body.

Some symptoms of depression may be relieved by such practices as:

- relaxation techniques—deep breathing, meditation, prayer, or hypnosis;

- exercise—yoga, Pilates, even walking 15 minutes a day;
- creative arts therapies—using dance, music, art, drama as outlets for emotional expression.

It is important for people with depression to receive professional help. People who rely on alternatives too much—who don't get treatment that is proven to be effective—can slip into a more serious depression that may be dangerous.

Length of therapy

Depending on how severe the depression is and the type of therapy chosen, psychotherapy may last just a few sessions or continue for several months. In general, the more severe or complicated the depression, the longer the time needed to treat it. Short-term therapy generally lasts for six to 12 sessions, while long-term therapy can last for months or even years.

PERSONAL AND SOCIAL SKILLS

Those who don't know how to develop and maintain friendships may become socially isolated. The Mayo Clinic (2003) reported that social isolation might contribute to depression. One way to avoid depression is by working with a professional therapist to improve communication skills.

SELF-ESTEEM

Self-esteem is the value individuals place on themselves. People with low self-esteem place little value on their abilities and achievement. Low self-esteem does not necessarily lead to depression but the two often go hand in hand. The Substance Abuse and Mental Health Services Administration (SAMHSA) notes that low self-esteem can be a symptom of depression. In addition, the Center for the Advancement of Children's Mental Health reports that people who have low self-esteem are prone to depression. Whether the links between the two are indicative of a psychological predisposition to or an early form of depression is not clear.

Communicating with friends, family, or the other people in one's life can be difficult for someone suffering from depression. Treatment for depression should include relearning communication skills such as **conflict resolution** and **self-disclosure** to help improve relationships. Conflict resolution is a set of skills that help individuals find peaceful solutions to disagreements. Self-disclosure is sharing information with others that they are not likely to know or discover on their own. Both communication styles involve risk and vulnerability on the part of those involved. Both may increase intimacy. Intimacy and closeness can help treat depression.

SOCIAL SUPPORT

The Mayo Clinic reported (2003) that having a social support network may help reduce the chances of depression. Social support is also important in dealing with emotional pain. Those suffering from depression should not be embarrassed to ask for help from family members or friends. Depression is an illness, not a personal weakness or defect in character. People who care about a person will want him or her to get help.

SCHOOL PROGRAMS

Most schools have a guidance counselor or therapist on staff. If your school does not, you can ask the school nurse for a referral. Some people with depression have concerns about confidentiality. Treatment for depression can only be successful if there is trust. Most professional counselors, nurses, and teachers recognize the importance of keeping conversations private.

Many students seek mental health treatment at school. According to SAMHSA, nearly 73 percent of the 83,000 public elementary, middle, and high schools that the agency surveyed for its report *School Mental Health Services in the United States, 2002–2003,* reported that social, interpersonal, or family problems were the most frequent mental health issues for both male and female students. Nearly one-fifth of students received some type mental health services in their school in the year prior to the study.

PROFESSIONAL
HEALTH-CARE PROVIDERS

Those who offer therapy and counseling services to the public often identify themselves by a confusing, long list of titles, including psychologist, licensed social worker, marriage and family therapist, psychiatrist, psychoanalyst, counselor, hypnotist, hypnotherapist, and psychotherapist. The most commonly used term is therapist.

In the United States, therapists are licensed by individual states rather than by the federal government. As a group, therapists encompass a wide variety of skill levels and approaches. People suffering from depression should seek a therapist whom they find intelligent, perceptive, and comforting. Finding a therapist who has graduated from a program recognized for its quality may be a good sign, but a degree from a prestigious university is no guarantee that a therapist is the right person for a particular patient. Similarly, many excellent practitioners are trained at lesser-known colleges and universities.

When considering a therapist or counselor, keep in mind a therapist is not meant to be a best friend or a substitute parent. A therapist is a professional who will help his or her patients heal themselves. People should not hesitate to "shop around" if they don't feel they've found a therapist who meets their needs.

Q & A

Question: I've been talking with my therapist about really intimate details of my life, and we've talked every week for a long time. Is it possible that we are becoming good friends?

Answer: Therapy is different from a friendship. A friendship is a two-sided relationship. Both people share their feelings. Although people often develop a close relationship with their therapist, therapy needs to be a one-sided relationship, one that focuses exclusively on the client's problems. By taking advantage of the unique relationship that develops in therapy, you are better able to make personal and emotional changes.

COMMUNITY AGENCIES

Almost every community has local organizations that can help those suffering from depression. Family or social services agencies, churches, and even organizations such as the YMCA or YWCA have connections to mental health professionals who can help treat depression. The United Way has a phone number that you can find in your local phone book (look under "First Call for Help" or "Information and Referral").

RATES

In 2003, the *Journal of the American Medical Association* released a study by the Harvard Medical School. According to the Centers for

Disease Control and Prevention, one in 20 Americans 12 years and older suffers from depression. In any two-week period, 5.4 percent of Americans in that age group experience bouts of depression, while depression rates were higher for women and non-Hispanic black people 40–59 years of age. Eighty percent of Americans who suffer from depression reported some level of impairment, while 27 percent reported that depression caused them to have serious problems at work.

The National Mental Health Association (NMHA) reports that of those who seek treatment for their depression, 80 percent show improvement. Too many people don't get treatment because they believe depression isn't serious, that they can treat it themselves, or that it is a personal weakness rather than a serious medical illness.

DEPRESSION IS TREATABLE

If you are depressed, you don't need to suffer with the disorder. Treatment is available and is likely to help you feel better. There are many places you can go for help. A number of local and national organizations offer professional help for people with depression. So do some schools. Friends and family may not always understand that depression is an illness, but relying on their support can be helpful both in avoiding depression and treating it.

See also: Depression, Symptoms of; Mental Health Professionals, Types of

FURTHER READING

Zucker, Faye, and Joan E. Huebl. *Beating Depression: Teens Find Light at the End of the Tunnel.* Scholastic Choices. New York: Children's Press, 2007.

HOTLINES AND HELP SITES

Active Minds
URL: www.activemindsoncampus.org
Phone: 1-202-332-9595
Programs: The young-adult voice in mental-health advocacy on more than 100 college campuses nationwide.
Mission: To provide peer-to-peer organizations dedicated to raising awareness about mental health among college students.

American Academy of Child and Adolescent Psychiatry (AACAP)
URL: http://www.aacap.org/
Phone: 1-202-966-7300
Address: 3615 Wisconsin Avenue NW
Washington, DC 20016-3007
Mission: Assist parents and families in understanding developmental, behavioral, emotional, and mental disorders affecting children and adolescents.

Alcoholics Anonymous
URL: http://www.aa.org/
Phone: 1-212-870-3400
Mission: To provide a fellowship of men and women who share their experience, strength, and hope with each other that they may solve their common problem and help others to recover from alcoholism. (Copyright © by The A.A. Grapevine, Inc.)

Anxiety Disorders Association of America
URL: http://www.adaa.org/
Phone: 1-240-485-1001
Address: 11900 Parklawn Dr., Suite 100
Rockville, MD 20852-2624
Mission: To promote the prevention, treatment and cure of anxiety
   disorders and to improve the lives of all people who suffer from
   them.

Codependents Anonymous (CoDA)
URL: http://www.codependents.org/
Phone: 1-602-277-7991
Address: Fellowship Services Office
PO Box 33577
Phoenix, AZ 85067-3577
Mission: To provide a fellowship of men and women whose common
   purpose is to develop healthy relationships.

Depression and Bipolar Support Alliance (DBSA)
URL: http://www.dbsalliance.org/
Phone: 1-800-826-3632
Address: 730 N. Franklin Street, Suite 501
Chicago, Illinois 60610-7224
Mission: To foster an understanding the impact and management of
   depression and bipolar disorder by providing information written
   in language the general public can understand. The organization
   also works to ensure that people living with mood disorders are
   treated equitably.

Families for Depression Awareness
URL: http://www.familyaware.org
Phone: 1-781-890-0220
Programs: Information and resources; family profiles, interviews
with people coping with depression; community outreach; awareness
workshops; advocacy.
Mission: To help families recognize and cope with depressive disorders to get people well and prevent suicide; to help families recognize and manage various forms of depression and associated mood
   disorders; to reduce stigma associated with depression; to unite
   families and help them heal in coping with depression.

National Hopeline Network
Phone: 1-800-SUICIDE (1-800-784-2433)
Mission: Toll-free, 24-hour crisis hotline.

National Institute of Mental Health
URL: http://www.nimh.nih.gov/
Mission: To research mental and behavioral disorders.

National Mental Health Association (NMHA)
URL: http://www.nmha.org/
Phone: 1-703-684-7722
Phone: 1-800-969-6642
Address: 1021 Prince Street
Alexandria, VA 22314-0297
Mission: To improve the mental health of all Americans, especially
the 54 million people with mental disorders, through advocacy,
education, research, and service.

Suicide Prevention Action Network (SPAN)
URL: http://www.spanusa.org/
Phone: 1-202-449-3600
Mission: To link the energy of those bereaved or touched by suicide
with the expertise of leaders in science, health, business, government, and public service to achieve the goal of significantly reducing the national rate of suicide.

GLOSSARY

acrophobia   severe and often debilitating fear of heights

addiction   a condition in which a person habitually gives into a psychological or physical need for a substance such as alcohol, tobacco, or drugs

Addison's disease   a disease in which the body does not produce enough of the hormone cortisol; can cause symptoms such as severe fatigue and muscle weakness, mimicking the symptoms of depression

adrenaline   a hormone secreted in the adrenal gland and produced in response to fear

aerophobia   also called aviophobia; fear of flying

agoraphobia   severe anxiety about being in open spaces or public areas; literally means "a fear of the marketplace"

anemia   a blood condition in which there are too few red blood cells

anorexia nervosa   a psychiatric diagnosis that describes an eating disorder, which is characterized by self-imposed starvation, low body weight, body image distortion, and an obsessive fear of gaining weight

antidepressants   medications that prevent or relieve depression

anxiety abnormal sense of fear, doubt about reality of the source of the fear, and self-doubt about coping with it

behavioral inhibition a tendency to react negatively to new situations or things

benzodiazepines drugs used to treat anxiety that work by slowing the activity of the central nervous system

beta-blockers fast-acting and non-habit-forming drugs used to calm anxiety symptoms such as shaking, palpitations, and excessive perspiration

bipolar disorder a brain disorder that causes unusual shifts in a person's mood, energy, and ability to function; also known as manic-depressive illness

blackouts loss of memory brought about by alcohol use

bruxism clenching or grinding of teeth

bulimia nervosa a psychiatric diagnosis that describes an eating disorder characterized by recurrent binge eating, followed by compensatory behaviors, referred to as "purging," or self-induced vomiting

cardiovascular relating to the heart and blood vessels

central nervous system the parts of the brain and spinal cord that control and coordinate most functions of the body and mind

checking an element of an obsessive-compulsive disorder that involves repeatedly inspecting or revisiting a previous action

chromosomes made of protein and DNA, a threadlike structure in cells that carries genetic information

chronic long-lasting or repeated

chronic pain   pain that lasts a month or more beyond the usual recovery period for an illness or injury, or pain that continues over months or years as the result of a chronic condition

circadian rhythms   rhythms of behavior that are associated with the 24-hour cycle of the Earth's rotation

cirrhosis   a disease that occurs when the liver is scarred so that it can't process and clean the blood as it normally does; often occurs as a consequence of alcohol abuse

claustrophobia   fear of enclosed spaces

cognitive behavior therapy (CBT)   a therapy based on the belief that pessimistic thoughts and negative views of life contribute to depression

cognitive distortions   mistaken beliefs or thoughts, usually about oneself

cognitive distortions theory   a theory based on the belief that depression and anxiety result from errors in thinking, such as jumping to conclusions, exaggerating the negative, and ignoring the positive

comorbid   refers to simultaneously occurring disorders or disorders that occur at the same time

compensation   a defense mechanism in which one part of the personality is stressed to make up for a perceived deficiency in another part

compulsions   uncontrollable urges to do something

conflict resolution   the process of resolving a dispute or a conflict by providing for each side's needs, and adequately addressing their interests so that they are satisfied with the outcome

conscious   awareness of the present

coronary artery disease   obstruction in the blood vessels leading to the heart

cortisol hormone produced by the adrenal glands and released in the body during stressed or agitated states

crack cocaine hard or flaky white rocks made from cocaine; intended for smoking

cultural values the standards, behaviors, or views that a society encourages

Cushing's disease an illness in which too much of the hormone cortisol is produced; can cause symptoms such as severe fatigue and muscle weakness, mimicking the symptoms of depression

delusions false beliefs held despite evidence to the contrary

dementia the loss of intellectual ability due to the destruction of brain cells

denial a defense mechanism used to avoid dealing with a painful reality

depressants drugs, including alcohol, tranquilizers, and inhalants (sniffers or huffers) that quiet and depress the nervous system

diabetes a disorder in which the body is not able to control its levels of blood sugar

diagnostic procedures tests or methods used to identify an illness or its cause

displacement a defense mechanism in which emotion is transferred from one subject or behavior to another less threatening subject or behavior

eating disorders psychological disorders, such as anorexia and bulimia, characterized by a compulsive obsession with food or weight

enabling behavior that that make it possible for someone with self-destructive behaviors to continue on without getting professional help

fight-or-flight response   the body's automatic and involuntary reaction to a frightening situation

flashback   memories of previous experiences that are vivid, realistic, and commonly frightening

gastritis   inflammation of the stomach walls

gastrointestinal system   a system of the body which includes the stomach and digestive tract; may respond to depression or anxiety disorders by speeding up or slowing down (nausea, constipation, or diarrhea)

gene   biological unit that directs production of a particular protein and determines the presence or absence of a particular trait

generalized anxiety disorder (GAD)   a mental illness consisting of more severe worry and tension than most people experience

genetic   inherited, shared genes give family members similar traits, such as hair color and eye color; genes are passed from parent to child

glucose   a form of sugar that provides the main source of fuel for the body

grief   great sadness or sorrow

group therapy   treatment in which a group of people meet with mental health professionals to talk with each other about how to deal with and resolve problems

hallucinations   false sights or sounds

hereditary   passed genetically from one generation to the next

HIV/AIDS   HIV is the retrovirus that causes the disorder that weakens the immune system known as AIDS (acquired immune deficiency syndrome). HIV destroys certain white blood cells and is transmitted through blood or bodily secretions

hormonal system the glands that secrete chemicals called hormones into the bloodstream to help the body cope with stress; also called the endocrine system

hormone a chemical substance produced to help the body's systems run regularly or grow

hypomania a less severe form of mania that does not impair a person's daily functioning

hypnosis a trancelike state of deep relaxation, relatively free of distractions; may be brought about by a therapist or by an individual for himself or herself

hypnotherapy the use of relaxation or hypnosis in treating illness, such as physical pain or mental disorders

hypoglycemia a physical disorder in which the body does not produce enough sugar

individual therapy a type of psychotherapy, often referred to as counseling, sometimes referred to as "talk therapy"

inpatient treatment psychological care as a patient in a health care facility

insomnia the inability to sleep

insulin a hormone produced by the pancreas that helps convert glucose to energy

interpersonal therapy a type of therapy that focuses on relationships as a way to understand and overcome symptoms of depression

introspection mental self-examination of feelings, thoughts, and motives

learned helplessness a theory based on the idea that helplessness is learned through experience with chronic or repeated stressful events

mania   part of bipolar disorder; elevated (high) mood or irritability accompanied by at least three of the following symptoms: overly inflated self-esteem, decreased need for sleep, increased talkativeness, racing thoughts, distractibility, increased goal-directed activity such as shopping, physical agitation, and excessive involvement in risky behaviors or activities

mass media   all of the communications sources that reach a large audience, especially television, radio, the Internet, newspapers, and magazines

menopause   the cessation of a woman's reproductive ability

mental disorders   psychological or mental states that can cause distressful effects ranging from mild sleep problems or relationship troubles to drug addiction or suicide

mitral valve prolapse   the failure of one of the valves of the heart—the mitral valve—to close fully after blood has passed from one chamber into another; can trigger symptoms of a panic attack

monoamine oxidase inhibitors (MAOIs)   antidepressants not commonly prescribed; interactions between MAOIs and other substances, including SSRIs, can cause dangerous elevations in blood pressure or other potentially life-threatening reactions

narcotic   a group of powerful, highly addictive drugs that relieve pain by preventing transmission of pain messages to the brain

neurotransmitter   a neurochemical, such as serotonin, that attaches to a receptor in the brain to transfer signals between a neuron and another cell

obsessions   unwanted, uncontrollable, and often inappropriate urges

obsessive-compulsive disorder (OCD)   a mental disorder consisting of distressing thoughts that don't go away and the repetition of certain behaviors or mental acts to cancel out these thoughts

obstructive sleep apnea a disorder that causes restricted and often interrupted breathing patterns during sleep

optimist a person who tends to feel hopeful and positive about life

ornithophobia a subtype of zoophobia; fear of birds

panic intense fear or anxiety that comes on suddenly, is overwhelming, and may seem to be unfounded

panic attack an episode of extreme anxiety that can include heavy perspiration, a feeling of suffocation, and strong and a rapid heartbeat

panic disorder a mental disorder diagnosed when a person has experienced at least two unexpected panic attacks *and* develops a persistent concern or worry about having further attacks or changes behavior to avoid or minimize such attacks

parasympathetic nervous system (PNS) the area of the nervous system that calms the body; works with the sympathetic nervous system (SNS)

perfectionist a person who is never satisfied with less than a perfect performance

pessimist a person who always expects the worst to happen

phototherapy bright light therapy

placebo a sugar pill with no medical value

post-traumatic stress disorder (PTSD) a mental disorder that may result from experiencing or witnessing a life-threatening event such as sexual, physical, or emotional abuse, military combat, a natural disaster, a terrorist action, a serious accident, or a violent assault like rape; symptoms include nightmares and flashbacks, difficulty sleeping, and feelings of detachment

predisposition   an increased likelihood that one will suffer from a particular disease

projection   a defense mechanism in which thoughts, feelings or impulses are unconsciously attributed to another person, especially if the thought or feeling is unwanted

psychedelic   type of drug that includes LSD, PCP, marijuana, and ecstasy; changes perception of reality (time seems to slow down or speed up; hallucinations and strange thought processes may occur)

psychiatrist   a medical doctor who specializes in mental, emotional, or behavioral disorders

psychoactive   having a profound or significant effect on mental processes

psychosis   a mental disorder that includes hallucinations and delusions

psychotherapy   the interaction between a therapist and a client to resolve symptoms of a mental disorder

puberty   the time of life when the sex glands begin to function

rationalization   a defense mechanism in which one tries to provide an acceptable explanation for a behavior or impulse that would otherwise be seen as offensive or objectionable

reaction formation   a defense mechanism in which someone unconsciously develops attitudes or behaviors that are the opposite of desires and impulses he or she find unacceptable

recidivism   the tendency to return to crime

repression   a defense mechanism in which a painful situation or fear is unconsciously excluded from the conscious mind

selective serotonin reuptake inhibitor (SSRI)   an antidepressant that acts on a chemical called serotonin, which helps the brain communicate with itself

self-disclosure   sharing information with others that they would not normally know or discover

self-esteem   one's opinion of oneself

self-talk   the things one says to oneself throughout the day

serotonin   a chemical that helps the brain communicate with itself

short-term memory   the part of the mind used to keep track of information for a brief period of time

social anxiety disorder   persistent, irrational fear of being in situations where one might be embarrassed; also known as social phobia

specific phobia   irrational, overwhelming fear of particular things

speed   an amphetamine that stimulates the nervous system

stereotype   an oversimplified generalization about a group of people

stigma   shame attached to something regarded as socially unacceptable

stimulants   drugs, such as caffeine, nicotine, amphetamines, or cocaine, that tend to increase alertness, energy, and physical activity

stress   emotional strain or discomfort felt from the pressures of life

subconscious   part of the mind below the level of awareness

sympathetic nervous system (SNS)   the area of the nervous system that revs up the body's system; balances the parasympathetic nervous system (PNS), which later calms the body

Tourette's syndrome   a disorder of the nervous system characterized by tics—involuntary, rapid, sudden movements or vocalizations that occur repeatedly in the same way

trance   state of relaxation in which attention is narrowly focused and relatively free of distractions

tricyclics   type of antidepressants that may cause side effects such as cause dizziness, drowsiness, dry mouth, and weight gain

trigger   event, feeling, or situation that precipitates other events or feelings such as a panic attack

uptake pump   a part of a communication system in the brain that reabsorbs serotonin after it is "sent" from a nerve cell, allowing more of the serotonin to be delivered to the "receiving" nerve cell

visualization therapy   form of self-hypnosis involving the development of a mental picture using all of the senses (vision, hearing, smell, touch, and taste); also known as creative visualization

vitamin deficiency   the lack of a particular vitamin in the body

vitamins   organic substances essential to nutrition and normal metabolism

zoophobia   the irrational fear of animals

INDEX

Boldface page numbers indicate extensive treatment of a topic.